Atlas of Transvaginal Endoscopy

Atlas of Transvaginal Endoscopy

Edited by

Stephan Gordts MD
Leuven Institute for Fertility and Embryology
Leuven, Belgium

and

Rudi Campo MD
Leuven Institute for Fertility and Embryology
Leuven, Belgium

Hugo Christian Verhoeven MD
Center for Reproductive Medicine and Endocrinology
Düsseldorf, Germany

Ivo Brosens MD PhD
Leuven Institute for Fertility and Embryology
Leuven, Belgium

With illustrations provided by

Patrick Puttemans MD
Leuven Institute for Fertility and Embryology
Leuven, Belgium

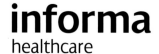

© 2007 Informa UK Ltd

First published in the United Kingdom in 2007 by Informa
Healthcare Ltd, 4 Park Square,
Milton Park, Abingdon, Oxon OX14 4RN
Informa Healthcare is a trading division of Informa UK Ltd
Registered Office: 37/41 Mortimer Street, London W1T 3JH
Registered in England and Wales Number 1072954.

Tel: +44 (0)20 7017 6000
Fax: +44 (0)20 7017 6336
Email: info.medicine@tandf.co.uk
Website: www.informahealthcare.com

Although every effort has been made to ensure that all owners
of copyright material have been acknowledged in this
publication, we would be glad to acknowledge in subsequent
reprints or editions any omissions brought to our attention.

A CIP record for this book is available from the British
Library.
Library of Congress Cataloging-in-Publication Data

Data available on application

ISBN-10: 1-84214-320-4
ISBN-13: 978-1-84214-320-9

Distributed in North and South America by
Taylor & Francis
6000 Broken Sound Parkway, NW, (Suite 300)
Boca Raton, FL 33487, USA

Within Continental USA
Tel: 1 (800) 272 7737; Fax: 1 (800) 374 3401
Outside Continental USA
Tel: (561) 994 0555; Fax: (561) 361 6018
Email: orders@crcpress.com

Distributed in the rest of the world by
Thomson Publishing Services
Cheriton House
North Way
Andover, Hampshire SP10 5BE, UK
Tel: +44 (0)1264 332424
Email: tps.tandfsalesorder@thomson.com

Composition by Scribe Design Ltd, Ashford, Kent, UK
Printed and bound in India by Replika Press Pvt Ltd

Contents

Contributors

Cristiana Barbosa MD
Florence Center of Ambulatory Surgery
Florence
Italy

Ivo Brosens MD PhD
Leuven Institute for Fertility and Embryology
Leuven
Belgium

Rudi Campo MD
Leuven Institute for Fertility and Embryology
Leuven
Belgium

Stephan Gordts MD
Leuven Institute for Fertility and Embryology
Leuven
Belgium

Sylvie Gordts MD
Leuven Institute for Fertility and Embryology
Leuven
Belgium

Caroline AM Koks MD PhD
Máxima Medical Centre
Veldhoven
The Netherlands

Emmanuel Lugo MD
Florence Center of Ambulatory Surgery
Florence
Italy

Per Lundorff MD
Viborg Hospital
Viborg
Denmark

Luca Mencaglia MD
Florence Center of Ambulatory Surgery
Florence
Italy

Ben-Willem Mol MD
Máxima Medical Centre
Veldhoven
The Netherlands

Carlos Roger Molinas MD PhD
Center for Gynaecological Endoscopy
Centro Médico La Costa
Asuncion
Paraguay

Patrick Puttemans MD
Leuven Institute for Fertility and Embryology
Leuven
Belgium

Hiroaki Shibahara MD PhD
Jichi Medical School
Minamikawachi-machi
Japan

Mitsuaki Suzuki MD PhD
Jichi Medical School
Minamikawachi-machi
Japan

Tatsuya Suzuki MD
Jichi Medical School
Minamikawachi-machi
Japan

Satoru Takamizawa MD
Jichi Medical School
Minamikawachi-machi
Japan

Yves van Belle MD
Kliniek Sint Jan
Brussels
Belgium

Olga EAA van Tetering EAA MD Mol BW MD PhD
Máxima Medical Centre
Veldhoven
The Netherlands

Hugo Christian Verhoeven MD
Center for Reproductive Medicine and
Endocrinology
Düsseldorf
Germany

Maarten AHM Wiegerinck MD PhD
St Joseph Hospital
Veldhoven
The Netherlands

Preface

Infertility is a complex disorder with significant medical, psychological and economic aspects. Both the prevalence of infertility and the number of patients seeking treatment of this disorder are increasing. With the introduction and the widespread use of assisted reproductive technologies (ART), the role of diagnostic laparoscopy in the evaluation of infertility has become controversial. Laparoscopy is invasive and expensive and is frequently omitted or postponed in the exploration of the infertile couple. The relative invasiveness of the standard endoscopic techniques and the increasing quality of the indirect imaging techniques are favouring this evolution, possibly resulting in a rather liberal referral to ART programs.

Up till now, however, direct visualisation of the different organs has proved to be superior to indirect imaging techniques. The easy vaginal accessibility of the uterus for hysteroscopy and the close contact of the tubo-ovarian organs with the posterior vaginal fornix make a trans-vaginal endoscopic approach tempting. Indeed cul-doscopy was the first technique offering the possibility of direct visualisation of the tubo-ovarian structures. The availability of small diameter endoscopes with high quality images offers today a minimally invasive way of access, enabling the accurate examination by direct visualisation of the reproductive pelvic structures, which was previously impossible. Both hysterosalpingography and diagnostic laparoscopy can be replaced by hysteroscopy and trans-vaginal hydrolaroscopy (TVL) as an ambulatory 'one stop fertility exploration'. In addition, TVL has been developed as a surgical tool in cases of ovarian capsule drilling in polycystic ovary syndrome, ovarian endometriosis and tubo-ovarian adhesions.

This atlas will show the reader the possibilities of the transvaginal approach in the exploration and, where possible and when indicated, surgical treatment of the uterus and tubo-ovarian structures.

Stephan Gordts

Section I

Diagnostic transvaginal endoscopy

1

Rationale of transvaginal laparoscopy in infertility

Stephan Gordts and Ivo Brosens

Introduction

Transvaginal laparoscopy (TVL) has been introduced as an alternative to standard laparoscopy (SL) for the exploration of patients with infertility. It is primarily a diagnostic procedure to be used in an office setting as a minimally invasive technique for the investigation of infertile patients with no obvious pelvic pathology. While SL is too invasive and probably not cost-effective to be performed in women without obvious pelvic pathology, the endoscopic exploration of the tubo-ovarian structures in infertility is in current practice frequently postponed or even omitted. As a consequence, diseases such as endometriosis, small endometriomas, or tubal disease are not diagnosed. However, even with the advent of in vitro fertilization (IVF) and the liberal referral to IVF we are not at the stage that we can ignore various uterine and pelvic pathologies associated with infertility, which may have an important impact on the reproductive outcome and can be corrected.

History

While attempts to use the transvaginal access for endoscopic exploration of the female pelvis go back to the beginning of the 20th century, the first successful technique of culdoscopy was introduced in the early 1940s by Decker.[1] The endoscopic visualization of the pelvic organs was performed with the patient in the knee-chest or genupectoral position. It was originally conceived as a complex hospital procedure with the patient in an uncomfortable and unstable position requiring elaborate mechanical and manual bracing and with the physician in an unusual physical orientation to the target organs. Small wonder that, when laparoscopy was introduced in the 1960s, transabdominal access was seen as the answer to some of the problems. Laparoscopy soon became the standard method for gynecologic endoscopy, particularly when it was shown that the technique was superior to culdoscopy for surgical procedures such as tubal sterilization.[2]

However, pioneers of pelvic endoscopy like Raoul Palmer[3] in Europe and Edward Diamond[4] in the USA continued to promote culdoscopy as the method of choice in at least one special application – the diagnosis of infertility, because it provides a closer, clearer, and more detailed view of the fallopian tubes, ovaries, and surrounding pelvic structures than laparoscopy. In 1978 Diamond[4] published a personal series of 4000 outpatient procedures of diagnostic culdoscopy in infertility. The results were impressive, the complications mild, and the failure rate was very low. Fimbrial phimosis and perifimbrial adhesions were more readily detected. Endometriosis could be seen on all the surfaces of the ovary, the distal end of the tube, the lateral pelvic wall, the utero-ovarian and uterosacral ligaments, and even in locations revealed with difficulty or not at all by laparoscopy. In particular, culdoscopy revealed the fine, filmy adhesions that are only rarely picked up by laparoscopy but which may be responsible for a significant amount of ovarian and tubal malfunction. Diamond concluded that the use of diagnostic culdoscopy as an outpatient procedure provides a better access for the diagnosis and treatment of infertility, especially when the pathology is not extreme enough to warrant laparoscopy. His advice was that the technique should be returned to gynecologic training programs, and he concluded:

> True, culdoscopy requires laboriously won special skills, but its advantage to patient and physician are well worth the trouble. Once mastered, culdoscopy equips the gynaecologic endoscopist with a rapid and minimally traumatic outpatient option that supplies rich information not only in the initial diagnosis of infertility but also in circumstances where laparoscopy might be inappropriate.

While the technology of laparoscopy has continuously improved, the technology of culdoscopy has not advanced since the 1960s. Improvements such as dorsal decubitus,[5] hydroflotation,[6] and miniculdoscopy[7] were suggested to revive culdoscopy, but received no further interest.

In 1998 Gordts et al[8] described a new culdoscopic technique, called transvaginal hydrolaparoscopy (THL), for the exploration of infertile patients without obvious pelvic pathology. A somewhat similar technique using a disposable cannula was developed by Watrelot and called fertiloscopy.[9] Both techniques combine the use of small-diameter instruments, dorsal decubitus, and hydroflotation.

Safety

SL requires general anesthesia and full operating room facilities. It is not an innocuous procedure, and the majority of laparoscopic complications occur during the transabdominal access.[10,11] One-third of the major complications are caused by the instillation of pneumoperitoneum and insertion of trocar.[12] Even in experienced hands, the bowel injury occurs as frequently during the access as during the surgical procedure and remains a major cause of morbidity and mortality.[13] In particular, the delayed diagnosis of bowel injury at SL is a major cause of sepsis and mortality.

The use of the small-diameter cannula and the combined needle trocar system in TVL add to the safety of the transvaginal technique. A large survey of transvaginal pelvic endoscopy reported that all bowel injuries were diagnosed during the procedure and supported the view that the small, non-leaking injury in healthy tissue can be managed expectantly without consequences.[14]

Underwater view

SL is not an ideal technique for the exploration of the tubo-ovarian structures in infertility. The panoramic view of the pelvis is obtained by distending the abdomen with CO_2 and by moving the bowels out of the pelvis using the Trendelenburg position and instrumental manipulation. While this panoramic view is essential in patients with major pelvic pathology or in acute conditions of pelvic pain or bleeding, it is very debatable whether the transabdominal approach and panoramic view of the pelvis are altogether needed for the exploration of infertility. The high intra-abdominal pressure during SL causes collapse of structures like the fimbriae and superficial lesions such as polypoidal endometriosis, filmy adhesions, and neoangiogenesis. In addition, the CO_2 pneumoperitoneum provokes pain with postoperative distress and induces acidosis, which is potentially harmful to the patient.

In transvaginal pelvic endoscopy the tubo-ovarian structures are directly accessible and the exploration is performed without additional manipulation. The aqueous distention medium keeps the organs afloat and enables the

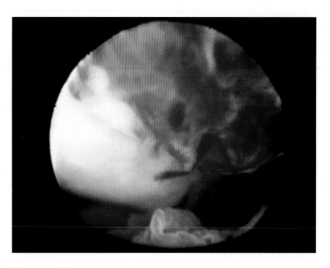

Figure 1.1
Cumulus mass capture by the fimbriae at the time of ovulation.

visualization of subtle tubo-ovarian structures in their natural position. The superiority of TVL over SL for exploring the tubo-ovarian architecture and physiologic processes, such as ovulation and ovum capture, was demonstrated when the first direct observation of the cumulus mass capture by the fimbriae at the time of ovulation was documented in the human[15] (Figure 1.1).

Hydroflotation and direct access to the fimbriae allows for accurate inspection of the fimbrial mucosal folds and the infundibulum by fimbrioscopy. Full salpingoscopy or ampulloscopy is more difficult, but can be achieved without additional instrumentation in approximately 50% of the patients, being most successful in the periovulatory period.[16] Salpingoscopy is not performed during SL in most centers because it requires training, is not an easy manipulation, and there is a need for an additional optical instrument and surgical assistance.

Finally, the use of an aqueous distention medium instead of CO_2 pneumoperitoneum avoids postoperative irritation and allows the patient to leave the office in comfort after the diagnostic procedure.

Accurate diagnosis

Mild and moderate pelvic lesions affecting fertility include peritoneal endometriosis, ovarian endometrioma, tubo-ovarian adhesions, fimbrial agglutination and phimosis, and tubal mucosal adhesions.

Endometriotic disease is today defined by the presence of any laparoscopically visible endometrial implant >5 mm, any visible ectopic endometrial implant with evidence of inflammation or tissue damage, such as neoangio-

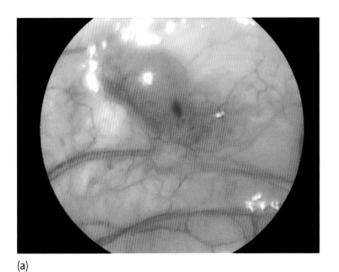

(a)

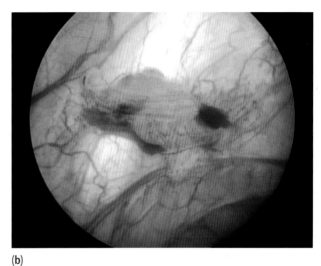

(b)

Figure 1.2
Effect of distention medium on appearance of peritoneal endometriotic lesion. (a) At standard laparoscopy using a CO_2 pneumoperitoneun, the lesion appears as a polypoidal implant. (b) The same lesion seen during transvaginal hydrolaparoscopy using an aqueous distention medium shows a free-floating, vascularized adhesion on a red hemorrhagic implant surrounded by intense neoangiogenesis.

genesis or adhesions without another explanation, or an endometrioma of any size.[17] For the accurate diagnosis we need a close and clear inspection of the lesion. Here, TVL offers major advantages over SL (Figure 1.2). First, endometriosis is frequently located at the caudal pole of the ovary and in the fossa ovarica. These locations are directly accessible at TVL. Without the need of supplementary manipulation, the whole ovarian surface and lateral pelvic wall can be inspected. Secondly, in mild and minimal endometriosis, 50% more ovarian adhesions are detected at TVL than at SL.[18] Small ovarian endometriomas, which are missed at transvaginal ultrasound, are detectable at TVL by the presence of superficial lesions, neoangiogenesis, and free-floating adhesions at the site of invagination of the ovarian cortex or agglutination of the ovarian gyri. Finally, endometriotic adhesions between the ovary and lateral pelvic wall, which may rupture and collapse during the manipulation of the ovary and appear as a diffuse bleeding at SL, remain intact. In conclusion, as women should not be considered to have endometriotic disease unless the ectopic endometrial implants show evidence of activity or tissue damage, we need accurate inspection of the lesion. Unfortunately, no recommendations exist under which conditions and by which criteria the tissue damage, inflammation, or neoangiogenesis should be evaluated and scored.

Fimbrial abnormalities and adhesions are also easily detectable at TVL. Studies of the fallopian tube in pelvic inflammatory disease have shown that the endoscopic inspection of tubal mucosa by salpingoscopy is the most accurate technique in predicting the probability of pregnancy and the risk of ectopic pregnancy.[19] In the presence of *Chlamydia* antibodies, exclusion of any tubal mucosal pathology is important for further fertility management.

Accurate diagnosis of uterine lesions, tubo-ovarian adhesions, and active peritoneal and ovarian endometriotic lesions at an early stage is important in the management of infertility. These lesions are assumed to affect 20–30% of subfertile patients. Capelo et al[20] found that one-third of the patients failing to conceive after four ovulatory cycles of clomiphene citrate had significant intrapelvic pathology. A multicentric study found that the performance of transvaginal endoscopy can mean avoiding laparoscopy in up to 93% of infertile women without clinical or ultrasound evidence of pelvic disease, as the relevant information can be obtained by this less-invasive procedure.[21]

Effective treatment

Endometriosis has been a major argument to opt for an endoscopy-based rather than ultrasound-based fertility investigation. The main question is whether minimal or mild endometriosis is a potential cause of delay in conception and whether surgical treatment is effective. A recent study of infertile women undergoing laparoscopy found that the time to natural conception differs significantly between women with unexplained infertility and infertile women with minimal or mild endometriosis.[22] In that study, a group of 192 fully investigated infertile couples were followed up for up to 3 years following laparoscopy. No surgical therapy was undertaken to treat the endometriosis found at that time. The authors found that the likelihood of pregnancy was significantly reduced in infertile women with minimal or mild endometriosis compared with those infertile women with a normal pelvis. Another recent study of 315 infertile patients with early-stage endometriosis and a control group of 152 infertile patients who had no endometriosis found significantly more fimbrial pathology, including agglutination, phimosis, and blunting, in the endometriosis group.[23] Clearly, in addition to the endometriotic lesions the presence of other mild pathology deserves endoscopic investigation.

The view that the diagnosis and treatment of minor endometriosis in an early stage of subfertility is beneficial is supported by the results of the Canadian Collaborative Group on Endometriosis.[24] In a study of 341 infertile patients with minimal and mild endometriosis who were randomized to laparoscopic ablation or expectant management, the authors found that laparoscopic ablation of minimal or mild endometriosis doubled the cumulative fecundity rate after a follow-up period of 36 weeks: 30.7% in the treatment group vs 17.7% in the no treatment group. A second Italian study could neither reject nor confirm this observation. The study included 101 infertile patients, but demonstrated no difference in fecundity rates after a follow-up period of 1 year.[25] A recent review combining the results of these two randomized controlled trials into a meta-analysis showed that surgical treatment is more favorable than expectant management (OR for pregnancy = 1.7; 95% CI 1.1–2.5).[26]

In a recent meta-analysis of IVF outcome for patients with endometriosis, Barnhart et al[27] recommended that patients with endometriosis of any stage should be referred for early aggressive infertility treatment, including IVF, to increase chances of conception. It remains an unfortunate fact that the diagnosis of endometriosis is still unduly delayed in many patients with infertility and pain.[28]

Timing the endoscopy-based investigation

The optimal approach in the management of female infertility requires that the timing and the method of the investigation are beneficial for the couple by avoiding both under- and overtreatment. Unfortunately, infertility is a disorder in which the diagnosis and, consequently, reliable treatments are frequently unduly and excessively delayed.

The duration of infertility, or the time to conception, has been used as a major parameter for timing routine exploration and starting treatment. It has been assumed that the longer the interval, the lower is the probability of conception, and therefore investigations should normally not start before 1 year of infertility.[29] On the other hand, a pro-

longed duration of infertility without preliminary endoscopic pelvic investigation has also been proposed as an indication for the use of assisted reproductive technology (ART). Therefore, in current practice, a delayed diagnosis may paradoxically favor both under- and overconsumption of ART.

Recent prospective studies on fecundity have shown that human beings may be more fertile than has previously been estimated.[30–32] In a recent debate Brosens et al[33] proposed that in view of the availability of less-invasive and more-accurate diagnostic tools and effective treatments, our current approach in timing the exploration of female infertility needs to be revisited. The issue is no longer when an invasive and expensive procedure like a laparoscopy should be performed, but at which stage a comprehensive minimally invasive fertility investigation is performed in order to inform the couple who worries about the delay in pregnancy. More than ever, the timing needs to be individualized, depending on factors such as age, medical, menstrual and sexual history, previous experience with contraceptive methods, use of fertility awareness methods for conception, and other individual factors. With the progress in minimally invasive exploration, the decision of timing the fertility investigation depends similarly as for other medical disorders in the first instance not on an abstract duration in time, but on the rational demand of the woman who worries about the cause of the delay of conception.

In older couples, some have argued that laparoscopy can be omitted from the infertility work-up when the hysterosalpingography is normal and there is no abnormal contributing history, and, as a consequence, the cost of fertility treatment is reduced without compromising success rates. However, Balasch[34] argued that in relatively older women an evaluation would find more diseases known to cause infertility, such as pelvic adhesions and endometriosis. Two studies aimed at determining infertility factors in women of advanced reproductive age concluded that there is no unique pattern of infertility diagnosis in such patients.[35,36] This supports the view that the routine investigation of infertility should not differ based on the age of the patient. Postponing the investigation in these women can be regarded as undertreatment when the couple is affected by a disorder or a combination of disorders for which an effective treatment, such as surgery or ART, may exist.

Conclusion

Today, the exploration of the female reproductive system, which traditionally included as the first step hysterosalpingography and at a later stage transabdominal laparoscopy, can be achieved in one step by minimally invasive transvaginal endoscopy. The procedure includes mini-hysteroscopy, transvaginal hydrolaparoscopy, fimbrioscopy, chromopertubation test and, in selected cases, salpingoscopy, and provides in a single procedure the most accurate and complete information on the reproductive organs. Therefore, transvaginal endoscopy is intended to replace hysterosalpingography as a first-line investigation, which avoids diagnostic laparoscopy in infertile patients without obvious pelvic pathology. The approach has the benefit of restoring in the infertile patient the normal stratification of a surgical procedure, which proceeds from diagnosis to full and accurate information of the patient, and of performing the surgical procedure after informed consent.

The clinical implementation of a new diagnostic tool, however, requires assessment of various aspects of the technique, including feasibility, safety, diagnostic accuracy, patient acceptability, and cost–benefit analysis. Several of these issues are discussed in detail in other chapters of this book.

References

1. Decker A. Culdoscopy – A New Technique in Gynecology and Obstetric Diagnosis. Philadelphia: WB Saunders, 1952.
2. McCann MF, Cole LP. Risks and benefits of culdoscopic female sterilization. Int J Gynaecol Obstet 1978; 16: 242–7.
3. Palmer R. Les Explorations Fonctionelles Gynécologiques, 2nd edn. Paris: Masson, 1974: 226–8.
4. Diamond E. Diagnostic culdoscopy in infertility: a study of 4,000 outpatient procedures. J Reprod Med 1978; 21: 23–30.
5. Mintz M. Actualisation de la culdoscopie transvaginale en décubitus dorsal. Un nouvel endoscope à vision directe muni d'une aiguille à ponction incorporée dans l'axe. Contracept Fertil Sex 1987; 15: 401–4.
6. Odent M. Hydrocolpotomie et hydroculdoscopie. Nouv Presse Méd 1973; 2: 187.
7. van Lith DAF, van Schie KJ, Beekhuizen W. Diagnostic miniculdoscopy preceding laparoscopy when bowel adhesions are suspected. J Reprod Med 1997; 23: 87–90.
8. Gordts S, Campo R, Rombauts L et al. Transvaginal hydrolaparoscopy as an outpatient procedure for infertility investigation. Hum Reprod 1998; 13: 99–103.
9. Watrelot A, Dreyfus JM, Andine JP. Evaluation of the performance of fertiloscopy in 160 consecutive infertile patients with no obvious pathology. Hum Reprod 1999; 14, 707–11.
10. Jansen FJ, Kapiteyn K, Trimbos-Kemper T et al. Complications of laparoscopy: a prospective multicentric observational study. Br J Obstet Gynaecol 1997; 104: 595–600.
11. Querleu D, Chapron C, Chevalier L et al. Complications of gynaecologic laparoscopic surgery – a French multicentre collaborative study. Gynaecol Endosc 1993; 2: 3–6.
12. Oshinsky GS, Smith AD. Laparoscopic needles and trocars: an overview of designs and complications. J Laparoendosc Surg 1992; 2: 117–25.
13. Brosens I, Gordon A, Campo R et al. Bowel injury in gynecologic laparoscopy. J Am Assoc Gynecol Laparosc 2003; 10: 9–13.
14. Gordts S, Watrelot A, Campo R et al. Risk and outcome of bowel injury during transvaginal pelvic endoscopy. Fertil Steril 2001; 76: 1238–41.
15. Gordts S, Campo R, Rombauts L et al. Endoscopic visualisation of

16. the process of fimbrial ovum retrieval in the human. Hum Reprod 1998; 13: 1425–8.
16. Gordts S, Campo R, Rombauts L et al. Transvaginal salpingoscopy: an office procedure for infertility investigation. Fertil Steril 1998; 70: 523–6.
17. Zondervan KT, Cardon LR, Kennedy SH. What makes a good case-control study? Design issues for complex traits such as endometriosis. Hum Reprod 2002; 17: 1415–23.
18. Brosens I, Gordts S, Campo R. Transvaginal hydrolaparoscopy but not standard laparoscopy reveals subtle endometriotic adhesions of the ovary. Fertil Steril 2001; 75: 1009–12.
19. Marana R, Catalano GF, Muzii L. Salpingoscopy. Curr Opin Obstet Gynecol 2003; 15: 333–6.
20. Capelo FO, Kumar A, Steinkampf MP et al. Laparoscopic evaluation following failure to achieve pregnancy after ovulation induction with clomiphene citrate. Fertil Steril 2003; 80: 1450–3.
21. Watrelot A, Nisolle M, Chelli H et al. International Group for Fertiloscopy Evaluation. Is laparoscopy still the gold standard in infertility assessment? A comparison of fertiloscopy versus laparoscopy in infertility. Results of an international multicentre prospective trial: the 'FLY' (Fertiloscopy-LaparoscopY) study. Hum Reprod 2003; 18: 834–9.
22. Akande VA, Hunt LP, Cahill DJ et al. Differences in time to natural conception between women with unexplained infertility and infertile women with minor endometriosis. Hum Reprod 2004; 19: 96–103.
23. Abuzeid M, Mitwally MF, Schwark S et al. A possible mechanical factor in infertile patients with early stage endometriosis. Fertil Steril 2005; 84(Suppl 1): S197.
24. Marcoux S, Maheux R, Bérubé S. Laparoscopic surgery in infertile women with minimal or mild endometriosis. The Canadian Collaborative Group on Endometriosis. N Engl J Med 1997; 337: 217–22.
25. Parazzini F. Ablation of lesions or no treatment in minimal-mild endometriosis in infertile women: a randomized trial. Hum Reprod 1999; 14: 1332–4.
26. Olive DL, Pritts EA. The treatment of endometriosis: a review of the evidence. Ann NY Acad Sci 2002; 955: 360–72.
27. Barnhart K, Dunsmoor-Su R, Coutifaris C. Effect of endometriosis on in vitro fertilization. Fertil Steril 2002; 77: 1148–55.
28. Dmowski WP, Lesniewicz R, Rana N et al. Changing trends in the diagnosis of endometriosis: a comparative study of women with pelvic endometriosis presenting with chronic pelvic pain or infertility. Fertil Steril 1997; 67: 238–43.
29. van der Steeg JW, Steures P, Hompes PGA et al. Investigation of the infertile couple: a basic fertility work-up performed within 12 months of trying to conceive generates costs and complications for no particular benefit. Hum Reprod 2005; 20: 2672–4.
30. Wang X, Chen C, Wang L et al. Conception, early pregnancy loss, and time to clinical pregnancy: a population-based prospective study. Fertil Steril 2003; 79: 577–84. .
31. Gnoth C, Godehardt D, Godehardt E et al. Time to pregnancy: results of the German prospective study and impact on the management of infertility. Hum Reprod 2003; 18: 1959–66.
32. Gnoth C, Godehardt E, Frank-Herrmann P et al. Definition and prevalence of subfertility and infertility. Hum Reprod 2005; 20: 1144–7.
33. Brosens I, Gordts S, Valkenburg M et al. Investigation of the infertile couple: when is the appropriate time to explore female infertility? Hum Reprod 2004; 19: 1689–92.
34. Balasch J. Investigation of the infertile couple in the era of assisted reproductive technology: a time for reappraisal. Hum Reprod 2000; 15: 2251–7.
35. Balasch J, Fábregues F, Jové IC et al. Infertility factors and pregnancy outcome in women above age 35. Gynecol Endocrinol 1992; 6: 31–5.
36. Miller JH, Weinberg RK, Canino NL et al. The pattern of infertility diagnoses in women of advanced reproductive age. Am J Obstet Gynecol 1999; 181: 952–7.

2

Diagnostic hysteroscopy

Rudi Campo and Carlos Roger Molinas

Introduction

Although operative hysteroscopy has progressively been accepted for the treatment of intrauterine pathologies, diagnostic hysteroscopy is still not widely and routinely used. Whereas almost all urologists utilize office cystoscopy to evaluate bladder pathology, it is estimated that less than 20% of gynecologists utilize office hysteroscopy to evaluate uterine pathology.[1] Conventional hysteroscopy, defined as a procedure performed with an instrument of 5.0 mm total diameter and with CO_2 as a distention medium and in which the insertion of the hysteroscope is facilitated by the use of a speculum and a tenaculum, has not been proven to be a technique accessible for all gynecologists and applicable in a routine set-up. Recently, well-conducted scientific studies have highlighted some important elements that can explain this underutilization of hysteroscopy as a first-line diagnostic procedure both in the office and in the conventional inpatient clinic. Nagele et al[2] have proved that CO_2 induces significantly more pain than a watery solution when used as distention medium.[2] Furthermore, a watery distention medium has the advantage of cleaning the environment, leading to a better and easier visualization of the uterine cavity than with the conventional CO_2. In a prospective randomized trial (PRT) we have recently proved the importance of the instrument diameter for both patient compliance and visualization quality.[3] In the same study we also demonstrated that both the experience of the surgeon and the anatomical difficulties determined by patient's parity play a key role when a conventional hysteroscope is used. With the use of a mini-hysteroscope, however, neither surgeon's experience nor patient's parity influence the results, offering a significant improvement for patient compliance and visualization quality. Office hysteroscopy is wrongly associated to a large extent with the disadvantages of conventional hysteroscopy and unfortunately many physicians, including gynecologists who do not witness the recent technical developments, believe that office hysteroscopy is similar to conventional hysteroscopy but performed in an office setting. In addition, the benefits of incorporating hysteroscopy as a first-line diagnostic tool for the investigation of abnormal uterine bleeding (AUB)[4,5] and infertility[6–9] are still not completely assumed by the medical community, whereas the lack of expertise to perform the procedure is evident.

The office approach for diagnostic hysteroscopy

In order to propose the systematic use of diagnostic hysteroscopy and to avoid the still well-established delay in indication, it is mandatory to perform the technique in the office, ideally at the same time as transvaginal sonography (TVS). The most important challenge for the office approach is to be able to perform the procedure with an acceptable patient compliance. This should not be underestimated, since many patients still prefer the inpatient approach, believing that it will be pain-free.[10] Several alternatives have been proposed for pain reduction during conventional office diagnostic hysteroscopy, but the results are inconclusive.[11–16]

The scientific evidence gathered over the last years and the major technical improvements in the manufacturing of high-quality small-bored scopes (minihysteroscopes) have provided an answer to the question of how diagnostic hysteroscopy should be implemented successfully in an office environment[2,17–21] (Table 2.1).

Instruments for office diagnostic hysteroscopy

Hysteroscope

While the diagnostic hysteroscopes used in the past had a total outer diameter of 5.0 mm, recent technical advances have allowed miniaturizing the instruments without compromising the quality of visualization. Today, two systems are suitable for performing hysteroscopy in the office:

Table 2.1 Diagnostic office hysteroscopy instrumentation

Hysteroscope:

• 30° rod lens optic	2.0 mm	2.9 mm
• Diagnostic single-flow sheath	2.8 mm	3.7 mm
• Operative single-flow sheath	3.6 mm	4.3 mm
• Operative continuous-flow sheath:	4.2 mm	5.0 mm

Additional instruments and maneuvers:

• Vaginal speculum	Not required
• Tenaculum	Not required
• Cervical dilatation	Not required

Distention medium: Low-viscosity fluids (e.g. saline) with pressure cuff between 80 and 120 mmHg

Analgesia/anaesthesia: Not required

- The mini-hysteroscope consists of a 2.0 mm 30° forward-oblique rigid telescope which fits in a single-flow examination sheath, leading to an instrument with a total outer diameter of 2.8 mm (Figure 2.1).
- The standard office hysteroscope consists of a 2.9 mm 30° forward-oblique rigid telescope assembled in a single-flow diagnostic sheath for a total instrument diameter of 3.7 mm (Figure 2.1).

Both telescopes can be inserted in a single- or double-flow operative sheet to transform purely diagnostic procedures to operative procedures. The total maximal instrument diameter increases for the 2.0 mm optic to 4.2 mm and for the 2.9 mm optic to 5.0 mm. In contrary to the diagnostic sheath the operative ones have an oval shape to reduce the instrument diameter as much as possible (Figure 2.2). The operative channel has an access for 5 Fr instruments, either

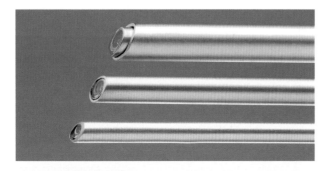

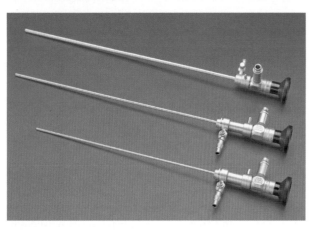

Figure 2.1
Comparison of diagnostic hysteroscopes of different diameter.

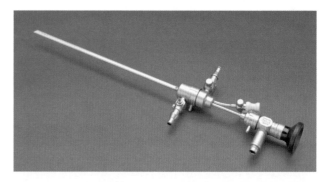

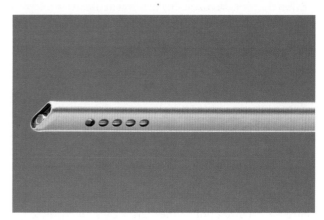

Figure 2.2
Operative hysteroscope.

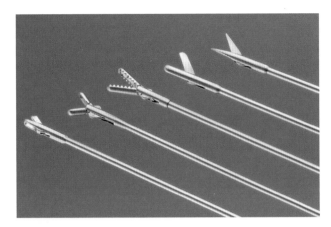

Figure 2.3
Mechanical instruments for operative hysteroscopy.

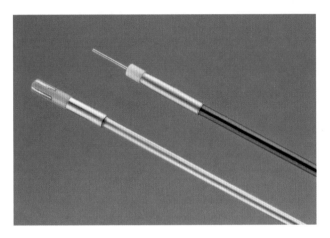

Figure 2.4
Electrical instruments for operative hysteroscopy.

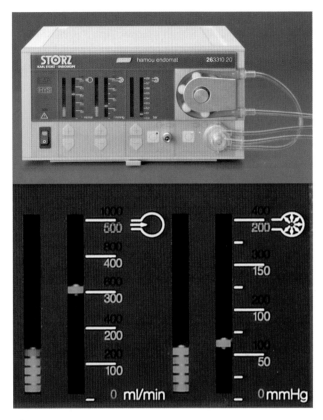

Figure 2.5
Electronic suction/irrigation pump.

mechanical (e.g. crocodile grasping forceps, spoon and punch biopsy forceps, sharp and blunt scissors, Figure 2.3) or electrical (e.g. bipolar needle, bipolar coagulation probe, Figure 2.4). This allows performing operative procedures in the office, such as visual guided biopsy, removal of small polyps, myomas or lost intrauterine devices (IUDs), and lysis of simple adhesions. The same instrumentation is used to perform the treatment of Asherman syndrome and the correction of congenital anomalies, but in those cases some form of pain relief is necessary.

Distention media

Since a good distention of the uterine cavity is required for performing hysteroscopy, the distention medium and the system to deliver it under certain pressure and flow must be

considered. For diagnostic hysteroscopy, either low-viscosity fluids with electrolytes (e.g. saline, Ringer's lactate, 5% glucose) or CO_2 can be used. To control pressure and flow, a simple gravity fall system, a pressure cuff, or an electronic suction/irrigation pump (Figure 2.5) can be used.

As a result of the differences in refraction index, fluid and gaseous distention media lead to different optical conditions. CO_2 is the most common gaseous distention medium used for hysteroscopy. The advantages of this natural gas are the good optical quality and, as a dry medium, its facility for use in an office environment. However, it must be supplied through a special pressure/flow-controlled unit to eliminate the danger of gas embolism,[22] it is limited to diagnostic procedures, and the current scientific evidence indicates that CO_2 is more painful and irritating than a fluid distention medium.[2] Mainly for the last reason, it is rapidly being replaced by fluid distention medium and is no longer used in many centers. The advantages of fluids lie in their simplicity, better patient compliance, and the excellent visualization capacity due to the rinsing and the hydroflotation (i.e. lesions floating in the watery low-pressure environment) effects. There is no blind phase at entering the cavity and no irritation of the peritoneum when the fluid enters through the fallopian tubes into the abdominal cavity.

For outpatient diagnostic hysteroscopy, an ionic, isotonic solution such as Ringer's lactate with a pressure cuff system is preferred owing to its cost-effectiveness and comfortable handling. The pressure cuff is mostly preset at a pressure between 80 and 120 mmHg, bearing in mind that the aim is to use the lowest-needed pressure to distend the uterine cavity correctly.

Light source

In 1960 Karl Storz discovered that it was possible to transmit light with fiberoptic light cables. This discovery marked the birth of cold light endoscopy. From a light source outside the body, light is transmitted via a fiberoptic light cable through an endoscope to the examination site. Only specific and particularly powerful halogen or xenon light sources are used in today's cold light projectors.

Video camera

The use of a video camera is essential for diagnostic hysteroscopic procedures. It is very instructive when the patient and the nursing personnel can see the diagnostic process on the screen and it is indispensable for correct documentation of the findings. Also, for the surgeon, the use of a camera facilitates the performance of the examination in a comfortable position.

Documentation system

The digital documentation systems AIDA (Advanced Image and Data Archiving) provide convenient image, video and audio data archiving of the procedure for academic and legal purposes.

Special office all in one solution, the TELE PACK system

TELE PACK is a comprehensive, multifunctional and compact documentation terminal that can be used as a compact system in the doctor's office, or as a secondary system in the operating room (Figure 2.6). It consists of the following components:

- *Input unit:* inbuilt, high-quality membrane keyboard and text generator for entering patient data.
- *Documentation:* flexible, all-purpose PCMCIA memory card for recording still images; easy transfer of data to AIDA and PC.
- *Camera control unit*
- *Illumination:* HiLux high-performance light source.
- *Image display:* foldaway LCD color monitor

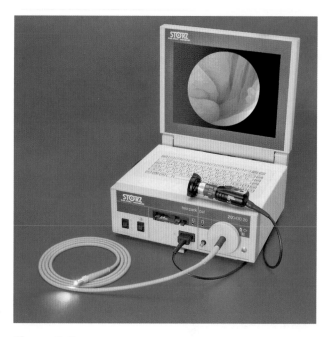

Figure 2.6
The TELE PACK system.

Technique

The use of mini-hysteroscopes and saline as a distention medium still allows approaching the uterus either with the classic technique, in which a speculum is used to visualize the portio and the external cervical os, or with the vaginoscopical approach, which we advocate. Because a speculum impairs the liberal scope movement, frequently leading to the necessity of using a tenaculum, we have adopted the vagino-cervico-hysteroscopy technique since the early 1990s. The examination is started with a TVS to evaluate uterus characteristics. A vaginal disinfection with a non-irritating watery disinfection solution is performed without placing a speculum. The tip of the hysteroscope is positioned in the vaginal introit, slightly separating the labia with the fingers. The vagina is distended with the same medium used for the uterine cavity. In contrary to the distention of the uterine cavity, the distention of the vagina does not provoke pain, even if the technique is not correctly performed. This approach requires a good knowledge of the physics and instrumentation as well as dexterity on the part of the operator (i.e. the correlation between what is seen on the screen and the actual position of the 30° fore-oblique scope). The scope is driven to the posterior fornix to readily visualize the portio, and slowly backwards to identify the external cervical os (Figure 2.7a). When this is visible, the scope is introduced into the cervical canal (Figure 2.7b) and, after achieving its distention, the scope is carefully moved forward to the internal cervical os (Figure 2.7c) and then to the uterine cavity with the least-possible trauma. The uterine cavity is systematically explored by

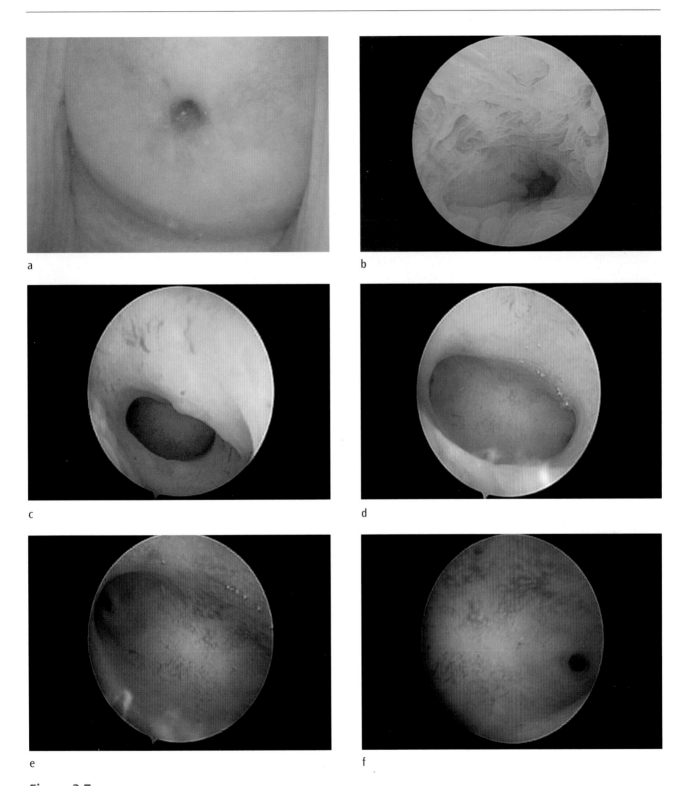

a

b

c

d

e

f

Figure 2.7
Hysteroscopy with the vaginoscopical approach. Visualization of the external cervical os (a), cervical canal (b), internal cervical os (c), uterine cavity overview (d), right tubal ostium (e), and left tubal ostium (f).

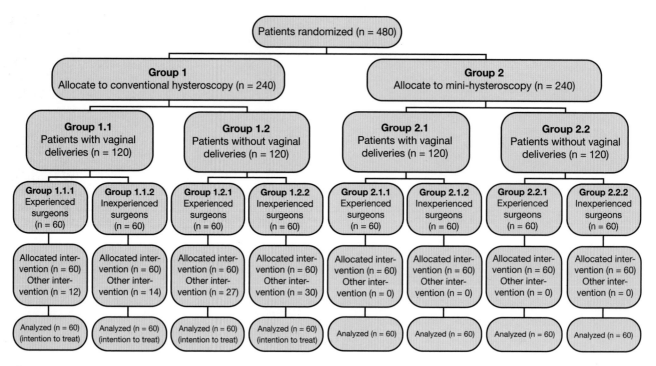

Figure 2.8
Prospective multicentric randomized controlled trial to evaluate factors influencing the success rate of office diagnostic hysteroscopy. Trial Profile. (Reproduced with permission from Campo et al.[3])

rotating the 30° fore-oblique scope and, after identification of the anatomical landmarks (i.e. the tubal ostia), any anomaly in the fundus, the laterals, anterior, or posterior uterine walls (Figure 2.7d) or in the right (Figure 2.7e) and left (Figure 2.7f) tubal ostium can be detected. At this stage it is crucially important to avoid lateral movements as much as possible to reduce patient discomfort to a minimum. Immediately after the hysteroscopy, a second TVS is performed, taking advantage of the intracavitary fluid for a contrast image of the uterus.

The importance of the instrument diameter and other factors in office diagnostic hysteroscopy

The advantages of the use of mini-hysteroscopes have been reported in many studies enrolling mostly patients with AUB and with previous vaginal deliveries.[19–21,23]

In an attempt to evaluate the effect of this (endoscope diameter) and other factors upon the success rate of diagnostic office hysteroscopy in a more general population we have recently conducted a PRT including 480 patients.[3] Together with instrument diameter (conventional hys-

teroscopy: 4.0 mm optic with 5.0 mm sheath or mini-hysteroscopy: 2.7 mm optic with 3.5 mm sheath), patient parity (with or without vaginal deliveries) and surgeon's experience (with or without experience in office hysteroscopy) were also evaluated (Figure 2.8). The following variables were assessed: pain (10 cm visual analogue scale: 0, none; 10, intolerable), quality of visualization of the uterine cavity (0, none; 1, insufficient; 2, sufficient; 3, excellent), and complication rate. From these variables, the success rate was calculated (pain <4, visualization ≥2 and no complications). Mini-hysteroscopy compared with conventional hysteroscopy was associated with less pain and better visualization, probably due to the less-traumatic passage through the cervical canal and the internal cervical os. The differences in visualization scores were only related to the quality of visualization of the uterine cavity rather than the quality of image itself, since it is obvious that the 4.0 mm optic provides a better image than the 2.7 mm optic. Although no differences in complication rates could be detected, probably due to the overall very low values, the success rates were higher with mini-hysteroscopy. In a multifactorial analysis, pain (Figure 2.9), visualization (Figure 2.10), and success rate (Figure 2.11) were highly influenced by instrument diameter and patient parity and only slightly influenced by the surgeon's experience. A better performance was observed with the use of mini-hysteroscopy, in patients with vaginal deliveries and in procedures performed by experienced surgeons.[3] The

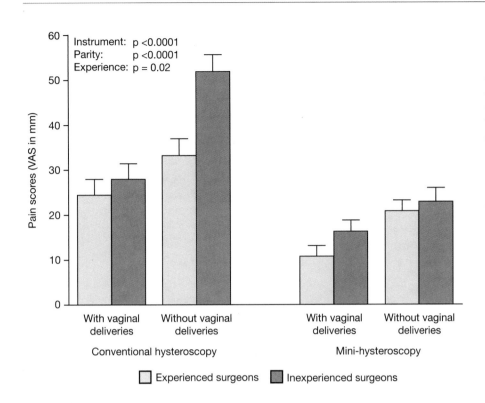

Figure 2.9
Effect of instrument diameter, patient parity, and surgeon experience upon the pain experienced by the patients during office diagnostic hysteroscopy. Pain was scored using a 10 cm visual analogue scale (0, none; 10, intolerable). The procedures were performed either with conventional instruments or with mini-instruments in patients with or without vaginal deliveries for experienced or inexperienced surgeons. Means ± SE, together with significances of a three-way analysis (proc GLM), are indicated. (Reproduced with permission from Campo et al.[3])

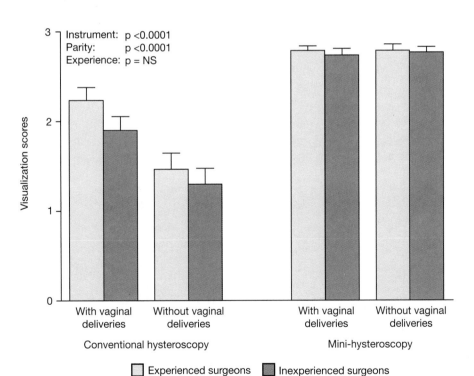

Figure 2.10
Effect of instrument diameter, patient parity, and surgeon experience upon the quality of visualization of the uterine cavity during office diagnostic hysteroscopy. Visualization was scored using a grading system (0, none; 1, insufficient; 2, sufficient; 3, excellent). The procedures were performed either with conventional instruments or with mini-instruments in patients with or without vaginal deliveries for experienced or inexperienced surgeons. Means ± SE, together with significances of a three-way analysis (proc GLM), are indicated. (Reproduced with permission from Campo et al.[3])

effects of patient parity and surgeon's experience were even more significant when conventional hysteroscopy was performed. This was not surprising, since in those patients and in those surgeons an easier access to the uterine cavity and less-traumatic maneuvers, respectively, can be expected.

Interestingly, both patient parity and surgeon's experience were no longer important when mini-hysteroscopy was performed, indicating that a small-diameter endoscope can counteract the difficulties determined by the anatomy and by the operator.[3]

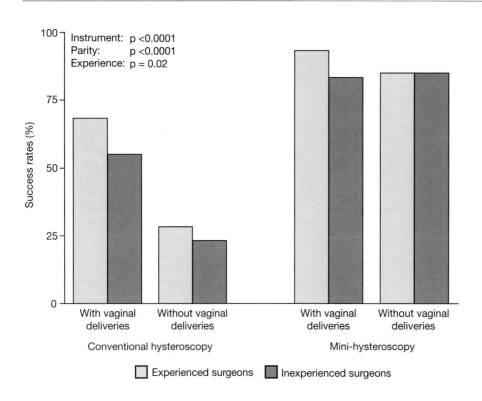

Figure 2.11
Effect of instrument diameter, patient parity, and surgeon experience upon the success rate of office diagnostic hysteroscopy. The procedures were considered successful when pain scores were <4, visualization scores were >1, and when no complication occurred. The procedures were performed either with conventional instruments or with mini-instruments in patients with or without vaginal deliveries for experienced or inexperienced surgeons. Frequencies, together with significances of a three-way analysis (proc logistic), are indicated. (Reproduced with permission from Campo et al.[3])

Indications for diagnostic hysteroscopy

The significant technical improvements in the field of hysteroscopy, including the use of mini-hysteroscopes, saline as distention medium, and the atraumatic insertion of the instruments, have allowed the performance of the procedure in the office and therefore broadened the indications for diagnostic hysteroscopy (Table 2.2). Indeed, office diagnostic hysteroscopy can be indicated today in any situation in which a major or minor intrauterine anomaly is suspected or necessary to rule out, including asymptomatic patients and for purpose of endometrial surveillance during drug treatment.

Table 2.2 Indications for office diagnostic hysteroscopy

- Abnormal uterine bleeding
- Infertility
- Abnormal findings at other diagnostic tests (e.g. ultrasound, hysterosalpingography, magnetic resonance imaging, blind biopsy)
- Repetitive pregnancy wastage
- Suspicious of uterine congenital anomalies
- Suspicious of intrauterine adhesions
- Misplaced foreign bodies (e.g. IUD)
- Follow-up of medical (e.g. tamoxifen) or surgical treatment
- Embryo evaluation (embryoscopy)

As with conventional hysteroscopy, the main indication for office diagnostic hysteroscopy remains the evaluation of AUB, including the suspicions of endometrial polyps, submucous myomas, and endometrial hyperplasia. Office diagnostic hysteroscopy is also indicated for the evaluation of the cervical and uterine factors in patients with infertility and especially in those who are scheduled to enter an in vitro fertilization (IVF) program. The time for this indication is the subject of continuous debate, since some clinics advocate systematic diagnostic hysteroscopy before IVF, whereas others delay the indication after several IVF failures. Other indications include repetitive pregnancy wastage, suspected intrauterine adhesions or uterine congenital anomalies, misplaced intrauterine foreign bodies (e.g. IUDs), reported abnormal findings at ultrasound, hysterosalpingography, magnetic resonance image or blind biopsy, and follow-up of certain treatments with intrauterine repercussions (e.g. tamoxifen or intrauterine surgery).

Furthermore, the already-mentioned simplification of the technique and the consistent data published over the last years permits us to propose office hysteroscopy as a first-line diagnostic tool for the investigation of AUB[4,5] and infertility.[6-9]

Controversial aspects and contraindications for hysteroscopy

Since the current technique of diagnostic hysteroscopy has decreased in trauma and manipulation, it is an intervention remarkably free of complications. There are no absolute contraindications, but still controversial questions are the dissemination of cells (e.g. germs, endometrium or cancer cells) into the abdominal cavity. In most cases during diagnostic hysteroscopy, distention medium floats through the fallopian tubes into the abdomen. This raises the question as to whether in case of inflammation of the vagina and/or the uterus ascending infections can occur thereafter or if endometriosis or peritoneal metastasis, in case of an endometrial carcinoma, can be promoted.

- An ascending genital infection after a diagnostic hysteroscopy is extremely rare and is not known in a series of several thousand hysteroscopies. Yet in cases of known vaginal or uterine infection the indication for a diagnostic hysteroscopy should be considered carefully and primarily the basic illness should be treated before a hysteroscopy is performed.
- As to the question of a potential furthering of an endometriosis, there are no available data with respect to diagnostic hysteroscopy. It can, however, be assumed that an inclination towards forming of an endometriosis follows different rules, especially as it is known that many women show retrograde blood and endometrium secretion during menstruation, but that only in a certain number of cases an endometriosis develops (autoimmune deficiency phenomenon?).
- Data about diagnostic hysteroscopy and spreading of tumor cells in cases of endometrial carcinoma are very limited. Several small studies did observe an increase of positive peritoneal cytology after fluid hysteroscopy. It is not known if this has any impact on the further course of the disease. To evaluate the influence of a diagnostic fluid hysteroscopy on the evolution of an endometrial carcinoma we only have available data of a comparable exam called the hysterosalpingography. Whereas this examination deliberately aims to transport the dye over the tubes into the abdominal cavity it is reassuring that the available data do not indicate any negative effect of performing this diagnostic procedure on the course of the disease. A still more important and as yet unanswered question is the possible effect of a dilatation and curettage (D&C) on the spread of carcinoma cells.

Active uterine bleeding, an absolute contraindication in the past, has become today only a relative contraindication since the use of continuous-flow hysteroscopy permits evacuation of blood and lavage of the uterine cavity, allowing visualization. Only profuse uterine bleeding remains as a real contraindication despite continuous-flow washing of the cavity.

Early pregnancy is not an absolute contraindication for hysteroscopy performed with the atraumatic technique described above (i.e. mini-hysteroscopes, saline distention medium, and vaginoscopical approach). Indeed, adverse effects have not so far been reported for hysteroscopy performed accidentally in early pregnancy. Furthermore, in case of intrauterine pregnancy with an IUD, it is recommended to remove the device because of the risk of abortions or septic complications. If the thread of the IUD is not visible, which often occurs because of growth of the uterus in pregnancy, it is advisable to extract it by either hysteroscopy or ultrasonic guidance.

As with any other diagnostic method, uncooperative or unstable patients, inappropriate training of the operator and lack of proper instrumentation also contraindicates the performance of the technique.

Complications of hysteroscopy

The possible complications of diagnostic hysteroscopy have been significantly reduced because of the smaller instrumentation and the less-traumatic technique. Nonetheless, even with these small instruments, complications such as uterine perforation, vasovagal reaction, laceration, and bleeding can occur. Campo reported 7 perforations in 4204 diagnostic hysteroscopies (0.16%).[24] No further problems occurred in these cases. Uterine perforation mostly occurs during introduction of the hysteroscope at the back of the uterus at the cervico-uterine junction. Conservative treatment is recommended and only in case of signs of inner bleeding in the following hours should diagnostic laparoscopy be performed. In a PRT involving 480 patients evaluating differences between conventional hysteroscopes (5.0 mm) and mini-hysteroscopes (3.5 mm), we found an overall very low complication rate (12/480, 2.5%), all of them being vasovagal reactions, whereas uterine perforation, cervical lacerations, or bleeding were not reported.[3] Interestingly, most of these complications were observed with the conventional hysteroscope (8/240, 3.3%) rather than with the mini-hysteroscope (4/240, 1.66%).

Findings at diagnostic hysteroscopy

All hysteroscopic findings are recorded in a standardized pre-design form. A complete visualization of cervical canal, uterine cavity, and tubal ostia and absence of any anatomical alterations is required to categorize the examination as normal. It is considered abnormal when any major or minor abnormalities, regardless of their clinical significance, are detected. If for any reason (i.e. patient tolerance, technical or anatomical problems) no or insufficient visu-

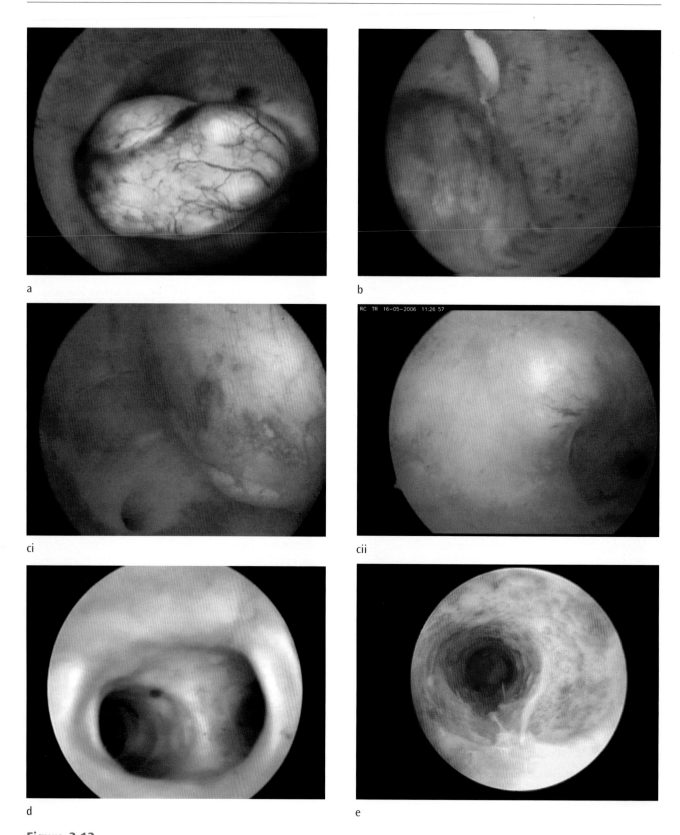

Figure 2.12

Major uterine abnormalities. Myoma with different degree of cavity involvement: (a) type 0, pedunculated; (b) type 1, intramural part but >50% in cavity; (c) type 2, major intramural part <50% in cavity. Congenital anomalies: (d) hysteroscopic image of a uterine septum; (e) hysteroscopic image by T-shaped uterus. Intrauterine adhesion and total obliteration of the cavity

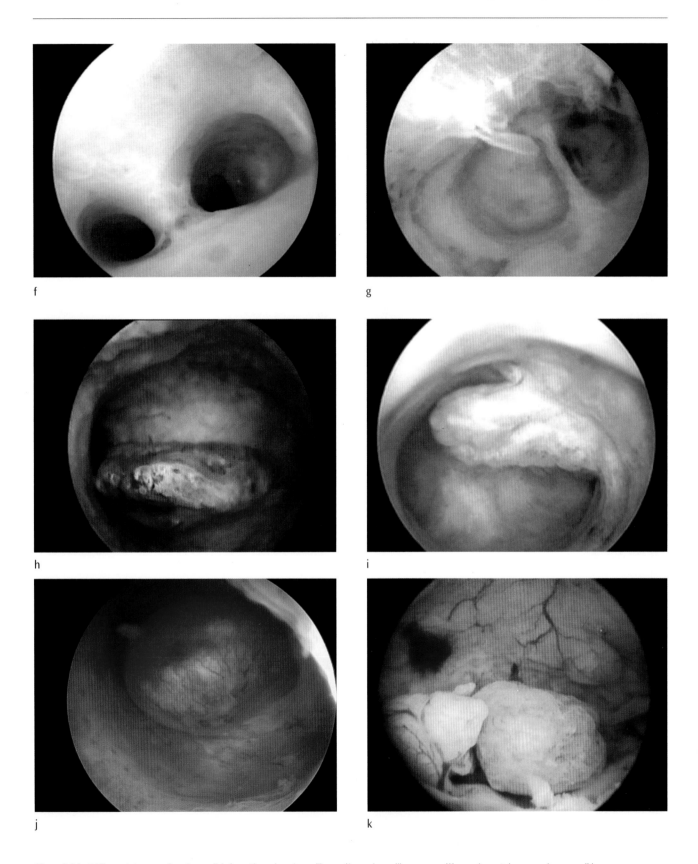

(f) and (g). Different types of polyps: (h) functional polyp; (i) sessile polyp; (j) myoma-like polyp. Adenocarcinoma: (k).

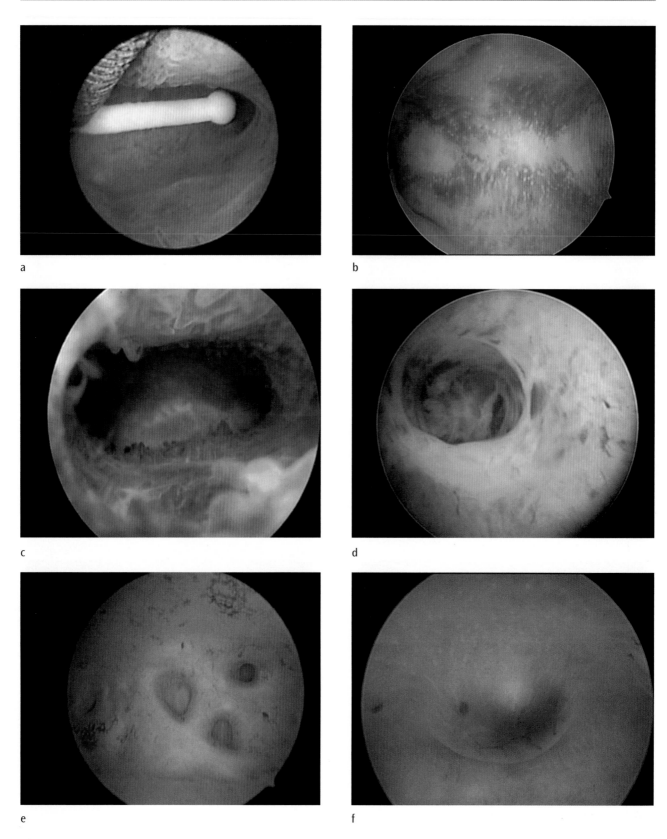

a

b

c

d

e

f

Figure 2.13
Hysteroscopic images of subtle lesions. (a) Hyperemic endometrium with intrauterine device. (b) Strawberry like pattern. (c) Diffuse polyposis. (d) Necrotic tissue (decidua). (e) Fundal endometrial defect (adenomyosis). (f) Moderate elevation, cystic lesion with a dark blue color originated from fluid blood in the lesion.

alization is obtained, it is stated that the examination failed to achieve a diagnosis.

- *Major abnormalities* are arbitrarily defined as those that structurally change the normal hysteroscopic anatomy (e.g. cervical stenosis, submucous myoma, polyps, congenital malformations, adhesions, necrotic tissue, tubal os stenosis, foreign bodies (Figure 2.12).
- *Minor abnormalities* or subtle lesions indicate changes of the appearance without deformation of the normal anatomy, where the pathologic significance is not always proven but where the hysteroscopic picture is different from the normal situation. These subtle or incipient lesions are described according to their hysteroscopic appearance and not to their supposed clinical significance (e.g. diffuse polyposis, hypervascularization, strawberry pattern, moderate/marked localized/generalized mucosal elevation (Figure 2.13).

In a recently published PRT we found that in the total population ($n = 480$) the findings were normal in 55% of the cases and abnormal in 41% of the cases, whereas no diagnosis could be obtained in 4% of the cases.[3] Interestingly, normal and abnormal findings were not equally distributed in patients with infertility or AUB. Indeed, in the infertility population ($n = 219$), the findings were normal in 67% of the cases and abnormal in 29% of the cases, whereas no diagnosis could be obtained in 4% of the cases. In the AUB population ($n = 230$), however, the findings were normal in only 46% of the cases and abnormal in 51% of the cases, whereas no diagnosis could be obtained in 3% of the cases. Furthermore, the specific findings were significantly different in both groups of patients (Figure 2.14, unpublished data).

Feasibility of diagnostic hysteroscopy

In the same PRT we found that the success rate, measured in terms of patient pain, visualization quality, and complication rate (see above), of diagnostic hysteroscopy was 65% (313/480). After discriminating by instrument diameter, however, this success rate rises to 87% (208/240) in the mini-hysteroscopy group and decreases to 44% (105/240) in the conventional hysteroscopy group ($p < 0.0001$). The mini-hysteroscopy was feasible for all assigned patients and, although the system included 3.5 mm and 2.4 mm scopes, the latter was necessary to use in five cases only (2%). For ethical reasons and to be able to obtain a diagnosis, the conventional 5.0 mm hysteroscope had to be changed to a mini-hysteroscope in 83 cases (35%; in 70 cases to a 3.5 mm scope and in 13 cases to a 2.4 mm scope), but patients remained in the assigned group for statistical

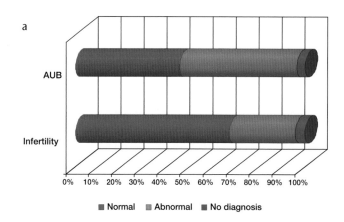

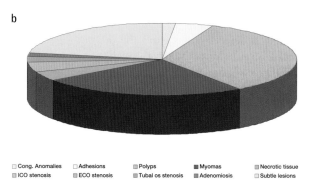

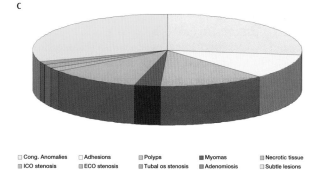

Figure 2.14
Hysteroscopic findings in patients with abnormal uterine bleeding (AUB) or infertility (unpublished data). (a) Distribution of normal and abnormal findings. (b) Abnormal findings in AUB patients. (c) Abnormal findings in infertility patients.

analysis (intention-to-treat). Since the smallest fiberoptic 2.4 mm hysteroscope was very seldom required, the data indicate that the rod lenses' 3.5 mm hysteroscope, combining the advantages of good optical quality and small diameter, is suitable for most cases.[3]

Conclusions

From the very first attempts at hysteroscopic diagnosis and treatment, starting with the examination by Commander Pantaleoni in 1869,[5] it was obvious that the inspection of the uterine cavity was not a simple technique. Problems related to light transmission, with bleeding from trauma of the very fragile endometrium and with the inability to distend properly the virtual uterine cavity surrounded by a thick muscular wall, slowed the development of hysteroscopy. Physicians convinced of the value of the technique had to focus on improving technical aspects and reducing instrument-related problems. Without ignoring the tremendous efforts made by pioneers of this technique, we have to acknowledge the fact that it was only in the last decennia that gynecologists, scientists, and engineers joined forces to develop instruments, as well as electronic and optical devices, that permit the diagnosis and treatment of intrauterine pathology through endoscopy, using a safe, atraumatic, and minimally invasive technique.

A major topic that has dominated this entire period of hysteroscopic research has been the improvement of safety measures during intrauterine procedures. Indeed, one of the major barriers to general acceptance of diagnostic hysteroscopy was caused by some lethal complications due to the use of inadequate CO_2 insufflation equipment. Based on experimental findings of the influence of CO_2 on the cardiopulmonary system, purpose-designed CO_2 hysteroflators that allow safe gas administration have been developed. Nowadays, however, distention medium for diagnostic hysteroscopy has changed in favor of using low-viscosity fluids (e.g. saline, Ringer's lactate) and the equipment required consists only of a pressure cuff, so that both risks and costs are very low. Together with the selection of the right distention medium, the miniaturization of the instruments plays a key role in intrauterine endoscopic procedures in an outpatient basis. The use of small instruments with outstanding optical features allows us to apply the atraumatic insertion technique in which the scope is introduced under visual control through the cervical canal, which is dilated only by the distention medium, into the uterine cavity, making it possible to obtain a perfect view of the endocervix and uterine cavity without any additional manipulation.

Diagnostic hysteroscopy, in combination with clinical examination and TVS, is a promising first-line diagnostic procedure in the gynecologic office to differentiate normal from abnormal situations. The endoscopic approach has, compared with the blind intrauterine manipulations such as D&C, the major advantage of permitting direct visualization of the pathology and selective treatment. For both major indications of hysteroscopy (i.e. AUB and infertility) this seems extremely important. For AUB patients, diagnostic and operative hysteroscopy offers an efficient organ-preserving technique. For infertile patients, diagnostic and operative hysteroscopy offers the possibility of preserving maximal chances for normal implantation and development of the pregnancy. Since the number of patients with infertility is constantly growing and the mean age of the infertile couples is increasing, the probability of intrauterine pathology is also growing. The scientific evidence on the success rate of office hysteroscopy and the reported incidence of intrauterine pathology after several IVF failures combined with the high cost of an IVF procedure makes it unacceptable not to implement diagnostic hysteroscopy in the routine exploration of the infertile patient.

In spite of the significant technical improvements, office hysteroscopy is still very poorly spread. Also, the recent scientific validation of the different parameters responsible for a simple, safe, and well-tolerated procedure has not led to a broad response. The most probable reason for the hesitation to implement office hysteroscopy is the lack of teaching at the majority of the universities during the residency in OB&GYN. In addition to the lack of teaching, the need to purchase endoscopic equipment often represents an important cost, which is not correctly reimbursed by most social security systems.

In summary, there is scientific evidence that the correct instrument selection, the atraumatic insertion technique, and the use of a watery distention medium are essential for successful office hysteroscopy. The miniaturization of the instruments opens the office procedure to inexperienced surgeons and makes it possible to offer this diagnostic procedure to the vast majority of the patients. Today, there is no clinical or scientifically acceptable reason for not implementing mini-hysteroscopy in daily practice as a first-line office diagnostic procedure in patients with infertility or AUB.

References

1. Isaacson K. Office hysteroscopy: a valuable but under-utilized technique. Curr Opin Obstet Gynecol 2002; 14: 381–5.
2. Nagele F, Bournas N, O'Connor H et al. Comparison of carbon dioxide and normal saline for uterine distention in outpatient hysteroscopy. Fertil Steril 1996; 65: 305–9.
3. Campo R, Molinas CR, Rombauts L et al. Prospective multicentre randomized controlled trial to evaluate factors influencing the success rate of office diagnostic hysteroscopy. Hum Reprod 2005; 20: 258–63.
4. Loverro G, Bettocchi S, Cormio G et al. Transvaginal sonography and hysteroscopy in postmenopausal uterine bleeding. Maturitas 1999; 33:139–44.
5. Cooper JM, Brady RM. Hysteroscopy in the management of abnormal uterine bleeding. Obstet Gynecol Clin North Am 1999; 26: 217–36.
6. Nawroth F, Foth D, Schmidt T. Minihysteroscopy as routine diagnostic procedure in women with primary infertility. J Am Assoc Gynecol Laparosc 2003; 10: 396–8.
7. Brosens I, Campo R, Puttemans P, Gordts S. One-stop endoscopy-based infertility clinic. Curr Opin Obstet Gynecol 2002; 14: 397–400.

8. Campo R, Gordts S, Brosens I. Minimally invasive exploration of the female reproductive tract in infertility. Reprod Biomed Online 2002; 4 (Suppl 3): 40–5.

9. Gordts S, Campo R, Puttemans P et al. Investigation of the infertile couple: a one-stop outpatient endoscopy-based approach. Hum Reprod 2002; 17: 1684–7.

10. Kremer C, Duffy S, Moroney M. Patient satisfaction with outpatient hysteroscopy versus day case hysteroscopy: randomised controlled trial. BMJ 2000; 320: 279–82.

11. Davies A, Richardson RE, O'Connor H et al. Lignocaine aerosol spray in outpatient hysteroscopy: a randomized double-blind placebo-controlled trial. Fertil Steril 1997; 67: 1019–23.

12. Nagele F, Lockwood G, Magos AL. Randomised placebo controlled trial of mefenamic acid for premedication at outpatient hysteroscopy: a pilot study. Br J Obstet Gynaecol 1997; 104: 842–4.

13. Wieser F, Kurz C, Wenzl R et al. Atraumatic cervical passage at outpatient hysteroscopy. Fertil Steril 1998; 69: 549–51.

14. Wong AY, Wong K, Tang LC. Stepwise pain score analysis of the effect of local lignocaine on outpatient hysteroscopy: a randomized, double-blind, placebo-controlled trial. Fertil Steril 2000; 73: 1234–7.

15. De Angelis C, Perrone G, Santoro G et al. Suppression of pelvic pain during hysteroscopy with a transcutaneous electrical nerve stimulation device. Fertil Steril 2003; 79: 1422–7.

16. Yang J, Vollenhoven B. Pain control in outpatient hysteroscopy. Obstet Gynecol Surv 2002; 57: 693–702.

17. Shankar M, Davidson A, Taub N, Habiba M. Randomised comparison of distention media for outpatient hysteroscopy. BJOG 2004; 111: 57–62.

18. Campo R, Van Belle Y, Rombauts L et al. Office mini-hysteroscopy. Hum Reprod Update 1999; 5: 73–81.

19. Cicinelli E, Schonauer LM, Barba B et al. Tolerability and cardiovascular complications of outpatient diagnostic minihysteroscopy compared with conventional hysteroscopy. J Am Assoc Gynecol Laparosc 2003; 10: 399–402.

20. Cicinelli E, Parisi C, Galantino P et al. Reliability, feasibility, and safety of minihysteroscopy with a vaginoscopic approach: experience with 6,000 cases. Fertil Steril 2003; 80: 199–202.

21. De Angelis C, Santoro G, Re ME, Nofroni I. Office hysteroscopy and compliance: mini-hysteroscopy versus traditional hysteroscopy in a randomized trial. Hum Reprod 2003; 18: 2441–5.

22. Lindemann HJ, Siegler AM, Mohr J. The Hysteroflator 1000S. J Reprod Med 1976; 16: 145–6.

23. Kremer C, Duffy S. A randomised controlled trial comparing transvaginal ultrasound, outpatient hysteroscopy and endometrial biopsy with inpatient hysteroscopy and curettage. BJOG 2000; 107: 1058–9.

24. Campo R, Van Belle Y, Rombauts L, Brosens I, Gordts S. Office mini-hysteroscopy. Hum Reprod Update 1999; 5: 73–81.

3

Transvaginal endoscopy: instrumentation and technique

Per Lundorff and Stephan Gordts

Introduction

As during the last decade improvements of the instruments have made optics thinner without losing the quality of the image, gynecologic endoscopy has changed and old techniques have gained popularity. Scissors, grasping forceps, and diathermy needles of 1 mm in diameter fitting into the 5 Fr working channels have proved their value. Using these smaller instruments, diagnostic procedures can become less invasive and the forgotten technique of diagnostic culdoscopy, a technique in which the endoscope is introduced through the posterior vaginal fornix,[1] can be re-evaluated.

The advantages of the transvaginal approach in infertility have been described in the French and English literature.[2-4] However, with the improvement of transabdominal laparoscopy and the possibility of performing laparoscopic operative procedures without a high risk of pelvic infections, the transvaginal approach was progressively abandoned. The high risk of sepsis associated with the culdoscopic approach was mainly due to the exteriorization of the Fallopian tubes.

With the patient in a dorsal decubitus position, the transvaginal endoscopy can now be performed in a minimally invasive way using a simple puncture technique of the pouch of Douglas and a watery solution as distention medium.

Instrumentation

To allow a safe and atraumatic entrance into the pouch of Douglas, a special needle dilator trocar system (Figure 3.1)

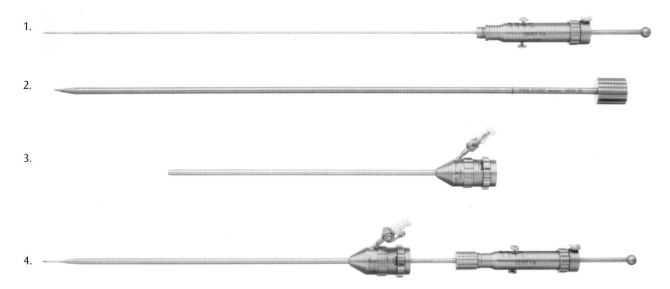

1.

2.

3.

4.

Figure 3.1
The specially developed needle trocar system allows easy vaginal entrance to the pelvic cavity by a simple needle puncture technique of the pouch of Douglas. To allow smooth transition from the needle diameter to the diameter of the outer trocar, the system consists of three parts: (1) the spring load needle, (2) the dilating device, and (3) the outer trocar with a diameter of 4.4 mm. The assembled system (4) is shown.

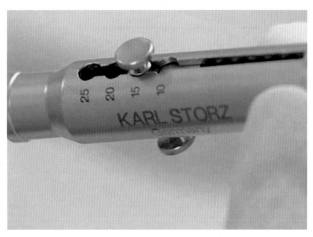

a

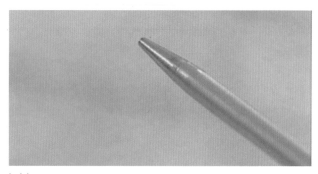

b (1)

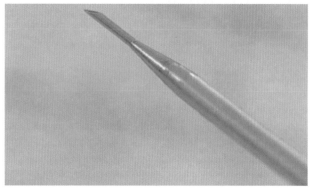

b (2)

Figure 3.2

(a) Springload needle with the possibility of presetting the length of the penetrating needle. Normally, a preset length of 15 mm is used. Only in obese patients can a longer length be indicated. The fast movement by firing the needle through the vaginal wall also reduces the pain sensation for the patient. (b) Point of the instrument before (1) and after firing (2) the needle with a preset length of 15 mm. Remark the smooth transition between the different parts.

(Karl Storz, Tütlingen, Germany) was developed to allow an easy access. The system consist out of three parts: (a) the springload needle, (b) the dilating sheet, and (c) the outer trocar of 3.5 mm.

The use of a springload needle makes access quicker and easier (Figures 3.2a and 3.2b).

The needle length can be preset between 10 and 25 mm. Routinely, the preset length is 15 mm and only in obese patients is the length extended up to 25 mm.

A 2.9 mm endoscope with a 30° angle lens and a diagnostic sheet of 3.7 mm is used both for hysteroscopy and transvaginal laparoscopy (TVL) (Figure 3.3).

Before use, the needle is passed into the dilating sheet (Figure 3.4). The unit is then inserted in the outer trocar and fixed with a counterclockwise movement.

In case it is indicated, this diagnostic trocar can be exchanged for an outer trocar with a working channel

allowing the insertion of a 5 Fr grasping or biopsy forceps and scissors. Changing from the diagnostic device to the trocar with the working channel is performed using a guide mandrin (Figure 3.5).

A light source, preferable a xenon light source, is necessary for illumination of the pelvic space. For obtaining documentation, a DVD recorder can be connected to the video camera. This recorder can store still pictures as well as minor video sequences.

An electronic pump unit system can be used for the hysteroscopy, but this is not mandatory for the TVL procedure, as filling of the pouch of Douglas can be obtained by gravity, connecting the irrigation bag directly to the flow channel.

The vaginal speculum has to have two open lateral sides, e.g. a Collin speculum, so it can be removed from the vagina soon after the placement of the outer trocar sheet.

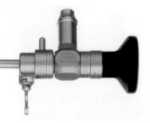

Figure 3.3

The 2.9 mm endoscope with a 30° angled optical lens inserted in the outer diagnostic trocar of 3.7 mm.

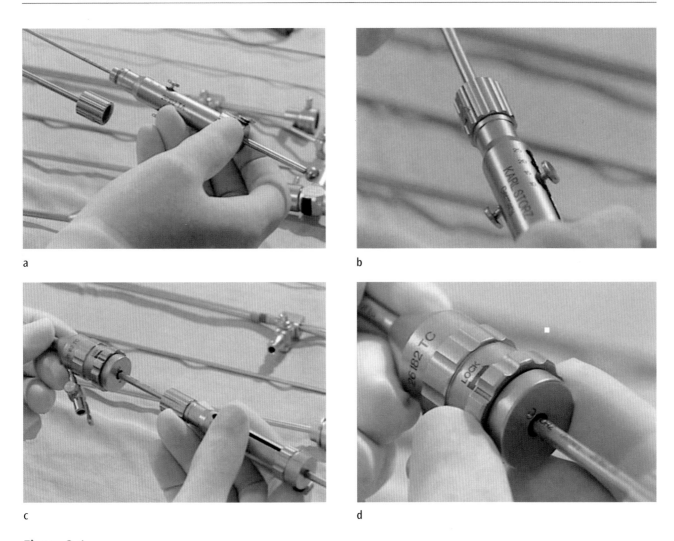

Figure 3.4
Assembling the system: (a) needle and dilating device; (b) needle is fixed by turning counterclockwise; (c) introducing assembled needle in outer trocar; (d) fixing outer trocar.

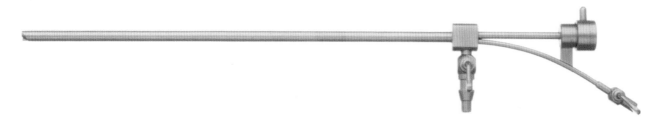

Figure 3.5
Operative outer trocar (5.6 mm) with one working channel allowing the use of 5 Fr instruments.

Technique

The transvaginal endoscopic exploration includes a diagnostic hysteroscopy and transvaginal laparoscopy performed in one session.

The patient is positioned in a dorsal lithotomy position. Prior to the procedure, a routine gynecologic examination and transvaginal ultrasound are performed to assess the size and position of the uterus and exclude contraindications for the procedure.

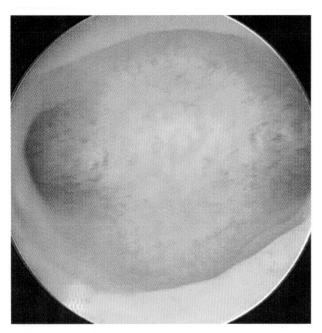

Figure 3.6
Diagnostic hysteroscopy using the 2.9 mm, 30° angled endoscope. Visualization of both tubal ostia becomes possible by turning the endoscope around its longitudinal axis.

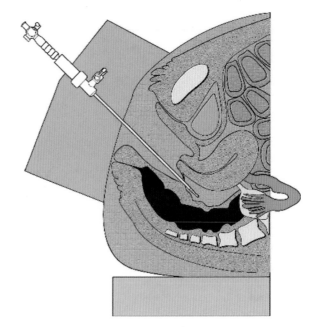

Figure 3.7
Using a specially developed needle-trocar system, access to the pouch of Douglas for performance of the transvaginal laparoscopy can be performed as a simple needle puncture technique of the posterior fornix about 1 cm under the cervix at the midline.

Hysteroscopy

After disinfection of the vagina with an aqueous solution of chlorhexidine, the examination starts with the mini-hysteroscopy, described by Campo et al.[5]

Without the use of a tenaculum forceps or speculum, the single-flow hysteroscope is introduced into the vagina under a continuous flow of Ringer's lactate at a pressure of 150 mmHg. or using an electronic pump system.

Cervical mucus can be helpful for easy identification of the external cervical ostium. The hysteroscope is then pushed slowly forward following the direction of the cervical channel. The dilating effect of Ringer's lactate solution facilitates the forward movement of the endoscope in the longitudinal direction of the cervical channel. Once the uterine cavity has been entered, the form of the cavity and the endometrium is inspected. Both tubal ostia and endometrium can now be easily visualized by rotating the endoscope around its longitudinal axis (Figure 3.6). Slow withdrawal of the endoscope allows easy exploration of the cervical channel.

Transvaginal laparoscopy

Patient selection

Diagnostic transvaginal laparoscopy is indicated in patients with subfertility problems or chronic pelvic pain without obvious pelvic pathology. The procedure has always to be preceded by a clinical vaginal examination and vaginal ultrasound with normal findings. Obliteration of the pouch of Douglas by large ovarian cysts or a fixed retroverted uterus are absolute contraindications, as are rectovaginal indurations or any acute situation such as bleeding or infection.

The procedure aims to evaluate the tubo-ovarian organs in their natural position and, wherever indicated, with patency testing, and to exclude the presence of adhesions and/or ovarian and pelvic endometriosis.

The procedure

Once the diagnostic hysteroscopy has been performed, the procedure of TVL can be started. TVL is performed either under sedation or using local anesthesia. During the entire procedure, a continuous flow of pre-warmed Ringer's lactate or saline is used to provide the abdominal distention and to keep the organs afloat. Access to the posterior pelvis is gained through a small needle puncture of the pouch of Douglas (Figure 3.7).

If performed under local anesthesia, the patients are able to follow the entire procedure on a video screen.

Using a dentist syringe with a 24 gauge needle the posterior lip of the cervix is infiltrated and consecutively grasped with a tenaculum (Figure 3.8), lifting up the cervix in order to expose the posterior fornix.

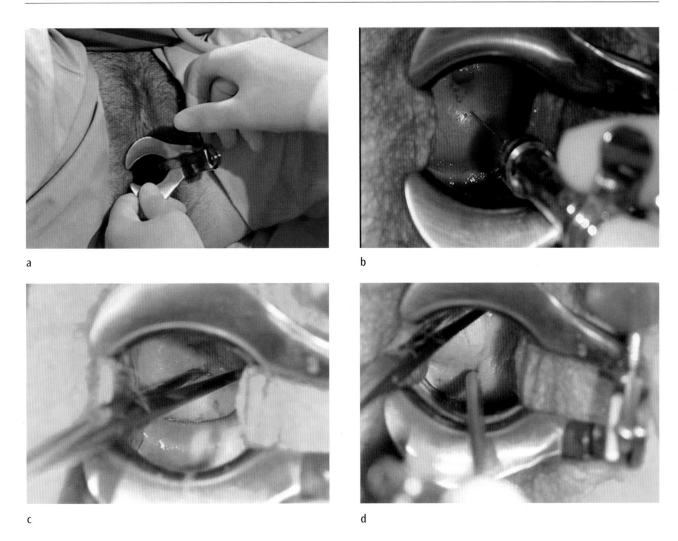

a

b

c

d

Figure 3.8
(a) Placement of a Collin speculum with two lateral openings. (b) Application of local anesthesia of the posterior lip of the cervix using a dentist syringe with 24 gauge needle. (c) Lifting up the posterior lip of the cervix with forceps; the bulbing of the vaginal wall is clearly visible (arrow). (d) Placement of assembled needle–trocar system on the midline at about 15 mm under the cervix.

Up and down movements show clearly the bulging of the vaginal fornix, which is helpful in identifying the point of entry. Subsequently, local anesthesia is applied to the posterior fornix.

The procedure can also be performed under sedation or general anesthesia in the operating room.

The assembled needle is placed at the posterior fornix on the midline about 1.5 cm under the cervix following the longitudinal axis of the vagina; this way, the needle will enter the pouch of Douglas between the uterine sacral ligaments (Figure 3.8d). The forceps, placed at the posterior lip of the cervix is lifted up and fixed with the left hand without traction (Figure 3.9). After the spring-loaded needle is placed at the right point, it is released. While fixing the forceps, the needle is slowly withdrawn while pushing the dilating sheet gently forward, followed by the insertion of

the outer trocar. The needle and dilating sheet are unlocked from the outer trocar and removed. Once the camera is mounted, the endoscope is introduced in the outer trocar to confirm a correct positioning of the instrument. For patency testing, where indicated, a Foley catheter No 8 can be introduced transcervically into the uterine cavity. The internal guide wire of this Foley catheter is helpful in passing the cervical channel. Once in the uterine cavity, the catheter is fixed by filling the balloon with 2 ml of saline, after the guide wire is removed. Once the instruments are in place, the forceps and speculum with open lateral sides are removed and the examination can be started. After verifying a correct intra-abdominal trocar position, the continuous flow of pre-warmed Ringer's lactate or saline is opened and the pouch of Douglas is filled with 200 ml, up to 500 ml. After the introduction of the endo-

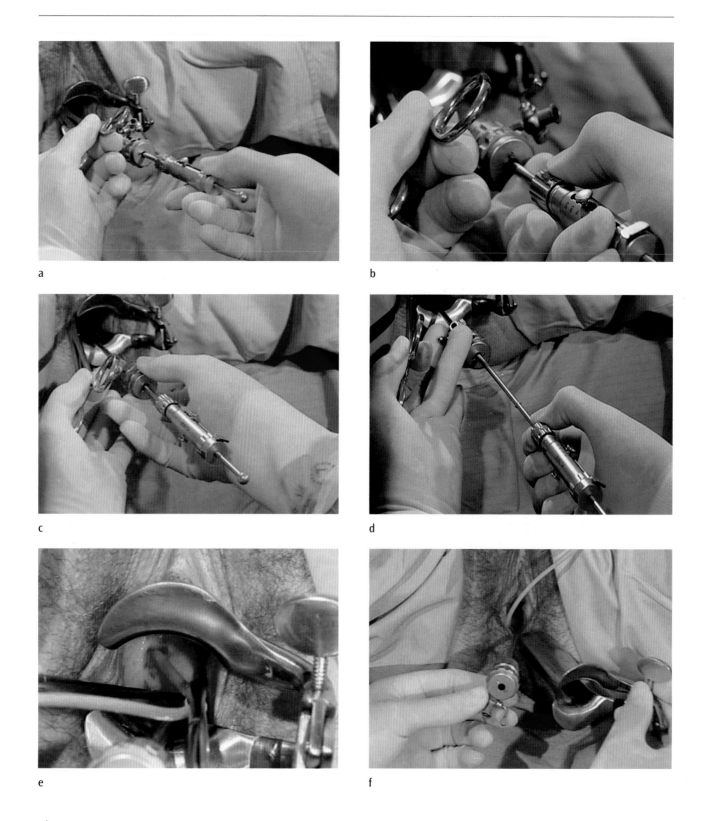

Figure 3.9

(a) After placement of the needle trocar unit at the right position, the springload needle is released by pushing with the thumb on the release button. (b,c) Once fired, the needle is gently withdrawn and the dilating device pushed forwards, followed by the outer trocar. (d) Removal of the needle and the dilator once the system is in place. (e,f) Placement of the Foley catheter No. 8 in case patency testing is required; because of the two lateral openings, the speculum can easily be removed.

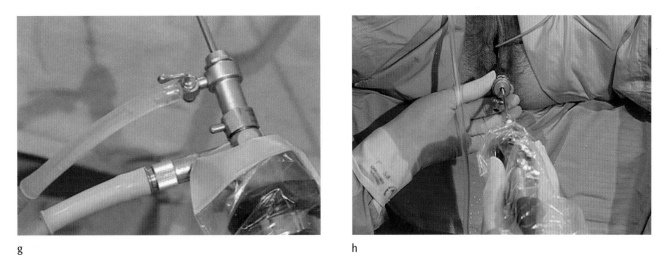

g   h

Figure 3.9 continued
(g) Connection of light cable, irrigation, and camera. (h) Positioning of hands during the procedure.

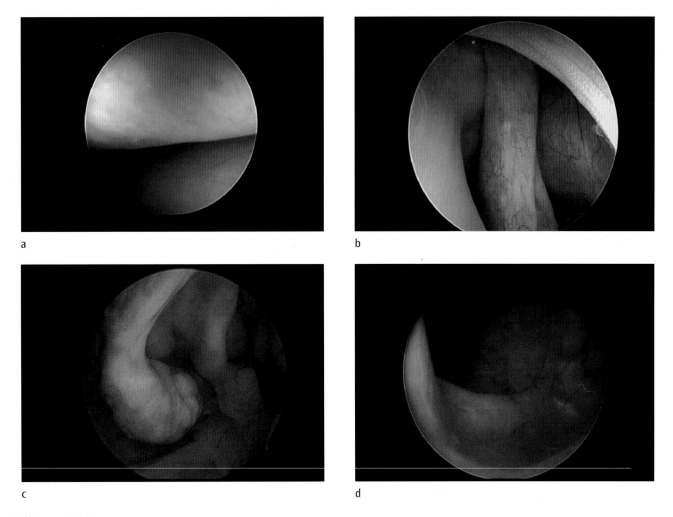

a   b

c   d

Figure 3.10
(a) In the absence of a panoramic view, the posterior wall of uterus is used as a landmark. (b) By rotation and lateralization of the endoscope and following the posterior uterine wall, the ligamentum ovarium proprium and isthmic part of the tube are identified. (c) View of ovary, ampullary part of the tube with free-floating fimbrial end. (d) By turning the 30° angled endoscope downwards, Douglas and sacrouterine ligaments can be inspected.

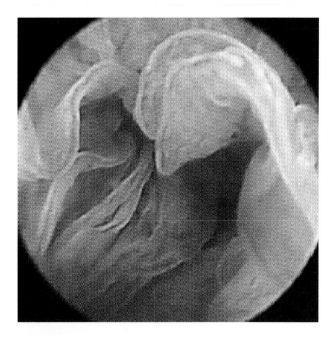

Figure 3.11
Whenever indicated, a patency test with methylene blue can be performed in conjunction with a fimbrioscopy and/or salpingoscopy.

scope, the posterior site of the uterus is looked for and, in the absence of a panoramic view, is used as a landmark (Figure 3.10). The procedure is performed as described by Gordts and Campo.[5,6]

Following the posterior part of the uterus, by rotation and lateralization, the ligamentum ovarium proprium and the isthmic part of the tube are identified (Figure 3.10b). The tube is followed downward to the fimbrial end. The entire surface of the ovary and the ovarian fossa can be explored by turning the 30° angled endoscope around its longitudinal axis, as in hysteroscopy (Figure 3.10c).

Moving back over the posterior side of the uterus, exploration of the contralateral adnexa is performed in the same way. Inspect the complete pouch of Douglas and the sacrouterine ligaments by pointing the 30° endoscope downward (Figure 3.10d). At the end of the procedure, a

patency test can be performed. While inspecting the fimbriae, the methylene blue can be gently injected. Having the endoscope in the longitudinal axis of the tubes and ovaries, salpingoscopy can be performed without further manipulation in approximately 50% of the tubes in which it is attempted.[7] Using a continuous flow, the endoscope can be introduced 1–2 cm into the ampullary part of the tube, allowing inspection of the major and minor mucosal folds (Figure 3.11).

At the end of the procedure, the endoscope is removed, and the used solution, normally between 200 and 400 ml of saline, is allowed to drain off through the cannula before withdrawal. The whole procedure is concluded by inspecting the posterior fornix for possible bleeding at the top of the vagina and posterior lip of the cervix. There is no need for suturing the puncture site unless active bleeding. The days following the examination, the patients can experience minor vaginal leakage and they are recommended not to use vaginal tampons, and to avoid coitus for 4–5 days. As the examination in the vast majority is performed as an outpatient procedure, the patients can leave the clinic immediately.

References:

1. Kelly JV, Rock J. Culdoscopy for diagnosis in infertility. Am J Obstet Gynecol 1956; 76: 523–37.

2. Palmer R. Les Explorations Fonctionelles Gynécologiques, 2nd edn. Paris: Masson, 1974: 226–8.

3. Diamond E. Diagnostic culdoscopy in infertility: a study of 4000 outpatient procedures. J Reprod Med 1978; 21: 23–8.

4. Mintz M. Actualisation de la culdoscopie transvaginale en décubitus dorsal. Un nouvel endoscope à vision directe muni d'une aiguille à ponction incorporée dans l'axe. Contracept Fertil Sex 1987; 15: 401–4.

5. Campo R, Gordts S, Rombauts L, Brosens I. Diagnostic accuracy of transvaginal hydrolaparoscopy in infertility. Fertil Steril 1999; 71: 1157–60.

6. Gordts S, Campo R, Rombauts L, Brosens I. Transvaginal hydrolaparoscopy as an outpatient procedure for infertility investigation. Hum Reprod 1998; 13: 99–103

7. Gordts S, Campo R, Rombauts L, Brosens I. Transvaginal salpingoscopy: an office procedure for infertility investigation. Fertil Steril 1998; 70: 523–6.

4

Normal tubo-ovarian events at transvaginal laparoscopy

Sylvie Gordts

Introduction

Transvaginal endoscopic exploration is intended to make the direct visual exploration of the female internal organs as minimally invasive as possible, without compromising the diagnostic accuracy of the endoscopic investigation. Although indirect methods for the exploration of the tubo-ovarian tract are commonly used as a first-line screening tool, direct endoscopic visualization of the uterine cavity and the tubo-ovarian structures is still considered to be the gold standard. Conventional transabdominal laparoscopy is too invasive for diagnostic purposes only, and therefore the exploration of the female pelvis is frequently postponed in patients with infertility. As a consequence, accurate diagnosis of disorders and appropriate treatment is therefore delayed or absent.

The transvaginal route offers direct and easy access to and visualization of the tubo-ovarian structures without supplementary manipulation. With the endoscope in the same axis as the adnexa, the whole ovarian surface and the ovarian fossa can easily be explored.

As pre-warmed Ringer's lactate is used as a distention medium, subtle lesions can easily be detected in their own natural environment. This is in contrast to the use of a high-pressure CO_2 pneumoperitoneum at standard laparoscopy, which will induce flattening and/or masking of subtle tubal and ovarian structures and lesions. A watery distention medium also keeps the organs afloat and will not cause peritoneal and diaphragmatic irritation like CO_2.

Since transvaginal laparoscopy can only be used in close contact with tissues and organs, and hence does not offer a panoramic approach to the female pelvis like conventional laparoscopy, it is important to have landmarks for one's orientation and to check the entire pelvis in a systematic way. Once the pouch of Douglas is entered, the optic has to be withdrawn and tilted upwards slightly to look for the posterior side of the uterus, the first landmark. Following the uterus up to the ovarian ligament and from this ligament down to the ovary, the whole ovarian surface and the ovarian fossa can easily be visualized subsequently. The whole length of the Fallopian tube can be followed, starting from its isthmic part down to the fimbrial end. When switching sides, one has to return to the starting point, i.e. to the posterior side of the uterus, and search again the ovarian ligament of the other side.

The posterior wall of the uterus

This is the place where the examination of the pelvis starts. This will also be the landmark for orientation. By following the posterior wall up to the fundus, one will reach the insertion of the Fallopian tube and ovarian ligament quite easily (Figure 4.1).

The ovary

By using an optic, angled at 30°, the whole surface of the ovary and the ovarian fossa can easily be visualized without any manipulation, except for the rotation of the optic itself. The ovary has a white surface, often with a recent or old ovulation stigma (Figure 4.2). During the follicular phase a pre-ovulatory or Graafian follicle can be visualized (Figure 4.3a).

It can happen that the ovary is lying more upwards, out of or even above the fossa ovarica. But by following the ovarian ligament, one should be able to find it quite easily without further manipulation. Sometimes, when the ovary lies in front of the uterus in the vesico-uterine pouch, a gentle manipulation with the optic might be necessary to dislodge the ovary from that position back to its normal location in the ovarian fossa. The word 'gentle' needs to be emphasized since that abnormal location may also be due

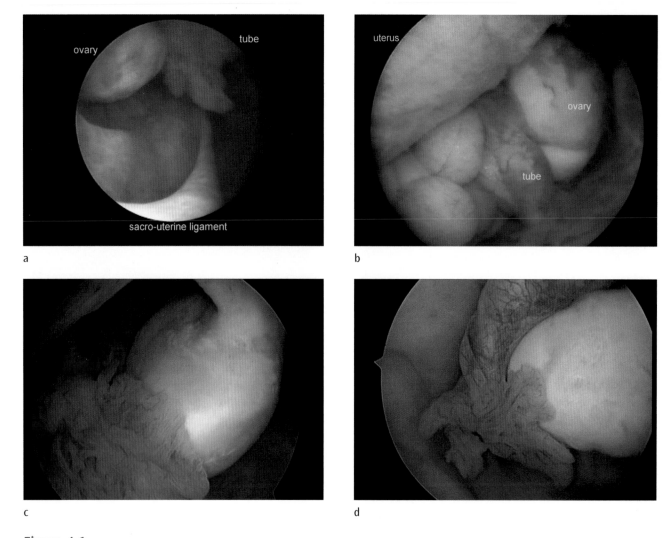

Figure 4.1
Normal anatomy.

to adhesions outside the visual field of the optic, fixing the ovary to the pelvic sidewall and/or uterus. In that case it is obvious that the patient then needs a standard laparoscopy.

The process of ovulation and ovum retrieval was observed endoscopically.[1] At the time of ovulation, the fimbriae on the ovulating side appeared congested and tumescent and showed pulsatile movements synchronous with the heartbeat of the patient (Figure 4.3c). The erect fimbriae were in close contact with the ovary, gently sweeping the surface of the ovulation ostium in a pulsatile way. On close inspection, a mucinous structure was seen protruding from the ovulation stigma, the fibrin threads of which were firmly adherent to the tips of the erect fimbriae. This mucinous structure was identified as the matrix of the cumulus–oocyte complex. The pulsatile movements of the fimbriae slowly pushed and pulled the cumulus–oocyte

complex free from the tear in the ruptured follicle. During the observation, follicular fluid leaked slowly out of the follicle. The total duration of the observation was 15 minutes. Erect fimbriae and pulsatile movements were not observed at the contralateral side. Apparently, vascular congestion causing erection and pulsatile movements of the fimbriae plays a role in the retrieval of the oocyte. The retrieval process from the site of rupture is slow, and active transport is achieved by ciliary activity of the tubal mucosa only. The fimbrial changes are apparently controlled by the ovulating ovary. A few days after the ovulation, a bridge between fimbriae and ovary can still be visualized as a mucoid web of fibrin threads (Figure 4.3d). Looking inside the ruptured follicle, the same weblike structure of fibrin threads can be observed, together with a yellowish colorization of the inside of the young corpus luteum (Figure 4.3b).

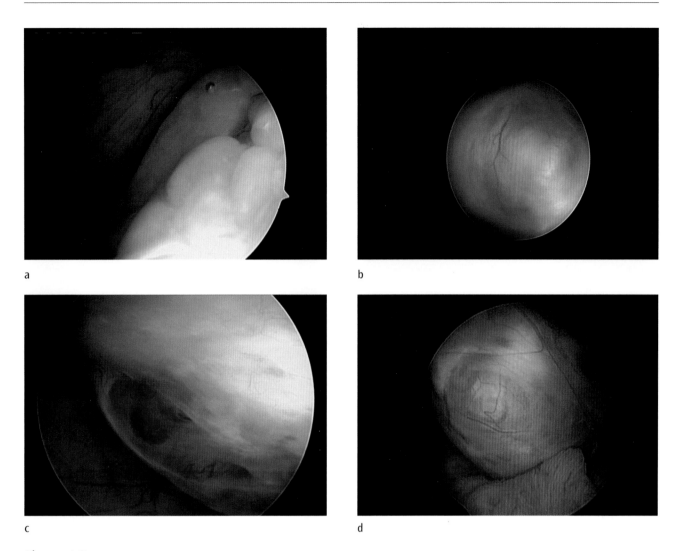

a

b

c

d

Figure 4.2
Normal ovary: (a) ovarian surface; (b) follicle; (c) fresh corpus luteum; (d) old corpus luteum.

Very often small white free-floating (i.e. non-adherent) or finger-like structures can be seen on the surface of the ovary (Figure 4.4). The importance of these findings has not been clarified so far. Pathologic examination of one of these lesions has shown a surface papilloma.

The Fallopian tube

Starting the exploration at its uterine origin, one can follow the whole length of the tube. The tubo-ovarian relationship can be inspected and tubo-ovarian adhesions can easily be seen. Nodular indurations at the isthmic level may rise the suspicion of salpingitis isthmica nodosa. The fimbriae can be visualized easily and should be free floating (Figure 4.1c and d).

Parasalpingeal cysts and hydatids and their relationship to the fimbriae can be observed in Figure 4.5.

Tubal patency

After examination of the whole pelvic cavity, tubal patency can be evaluated using dye injection through a uterine catheter. Even a strongly diluted solution of methylene blue might blur the vision, and therefore this part of the procedure needs to be done at the end. Even by using very little pressure, some filling of the tube and methylene blue leaking can be seen quite instantaneously.

Using this blue as a guide, it is often possible to perform a salpingoscopy without any further manipulation of the

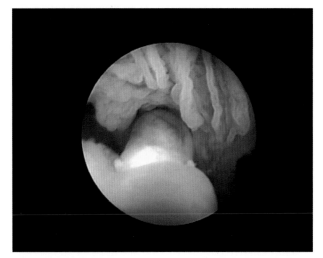

a

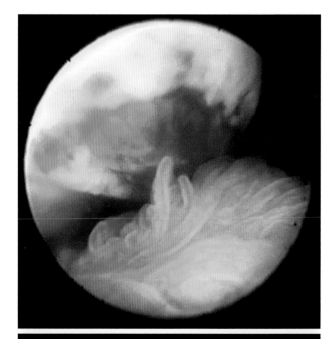

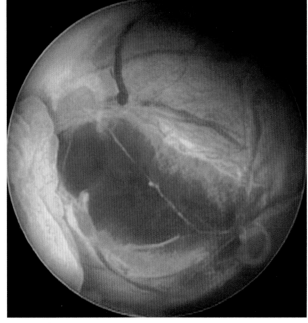

b

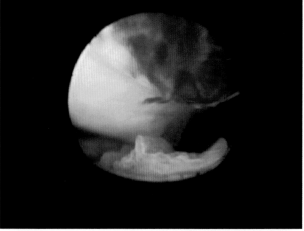

c

Figure 4.3

Events around ovulation. (a) Preovulatory follicle. (b) Fresh corpus luteum. (c) Erected fimbriae underlying the caudal pole of the ovary and sweeping the ovarian surface; presence of mucinous band (arrow) stretched between fimbrial ends and ovulation ostium. (Reproduced from Gordts et al. Hum Reprod 1998; 13: 1425–8[1] with permission from Oxford University Press.) (d) Postovulation mucinous web.

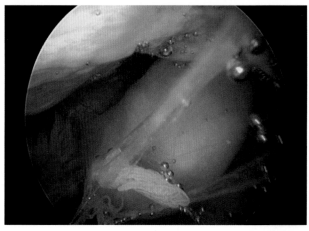

d

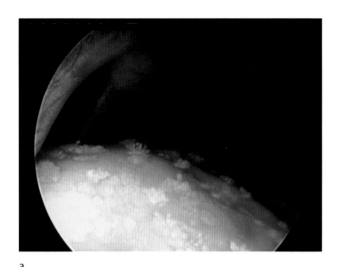

a

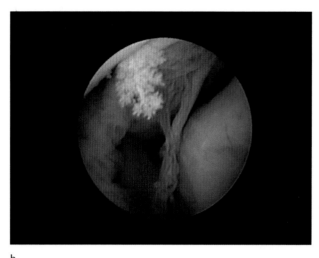

b

Figure 4.4
Small white adhesions on surface of ovary compatible at histologic examination with papilloma.

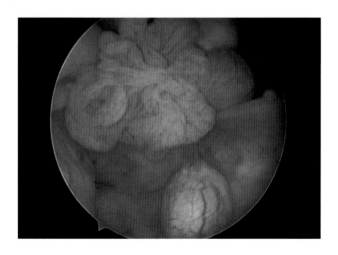

Figure 4.5
Parasalpingeal cyst.

tube (Figure 4.6). This can give an impression of the quality of the tubal mucosa and its folds in the ampullary part of the Fallopian tube up to the isthmo-ampullary junction (3–5 cm). Salpingoscopic findings can be classified, as described by Puttemans et al:[2]

- Grade I: normal mucosal folds are observed.
- Grade II: the major folds are separated and flattened, but otherwise normal (in fact, this might be considered a grade I tube, distended by an increased intraluminal hydrostatic pressure and therefore considered as normal, since these changes are reversible once that overpressure is eliminated, e.g. by opening a thin-walled but otherwise undamaged hydrosalpinx).
- Grade III: focal adhesions between the mucosal folds are seen.

- Grade IV: extensive adhesions between the mucosal folds and/or disseminated nude areas are present.
- Grade V: the mucosal fold pattern is completely lost.

Uterosacral ligaments and pouch of Douglas

Below the ovarian fossa, by turning the 30° optic upside down, one can visualize the uterosacral ligament and the peritoneal surface of the pouch of Douglas (Figure 4.1a).

The evaluation by transvaginal laparoscopy can be considered as complete when the posterior wall of the uterus, the ovaries – including their fossa – from all sides, the Fallopian tubes and their fimbrial ends, the uterosacral liga-

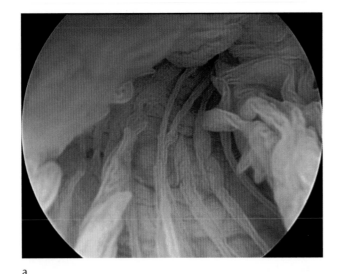

a

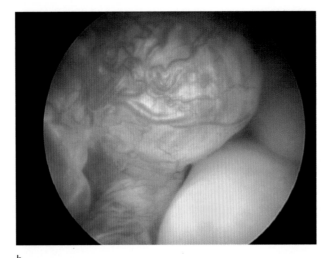

b

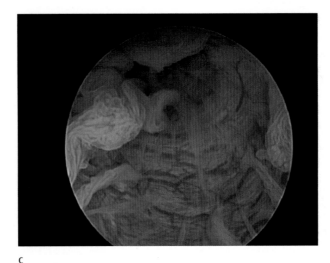

c

Figure 4.6
Salpingoscopy: (a) normal fimbrial folds; (b) hypoplastic tube, showing the thin muscular wall, and at salpingoscopy, the distended folds (c).

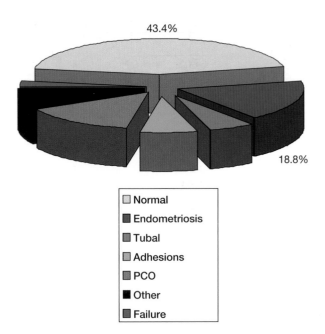

43.4%

18.8%

☐ Normal
■ Endometriosis
☐ Tubal
☐ Adhesions
☐ PCO
■ Other
■ Failure

Figure 4.7
Findings of 880 transvaginal laporoscopies.

ments and the pouch of Douglas are all visible and thoroughly inspected.

In the period 1997–2005 we performed 880 transvaginal laparoscopy procedures in infertile patients without obvious pathology. In 43.4% of patients, findings were completely normal. Endometriosis was found in 18.9%, tubal pathology in 5.5%, adhesions in 7.4%, and polycystic ovaries in 14.2% of patients. The failure rate was 2.8% (Figure 4.7).

Several studies have evaluated the accuracy of transvaginal laparoscopy.

The first study[3] was a prospective, comparative study including 10 infertile patients. It was found that transvaginal hydrolaparoscopy is comparable in accuracy to standard laparoscopy for the diagnosis of adhesions and endometriosis in infertile patients without obvious pathology.

The study of Darai et al[4] was a prospective blind study, including 60 infertile patients, not excluding women with prior pelvic or abdominal surgery. It was found that only 44.5% of the patients had normal pelvic findings. The ability to evaluate the pelvis and its structures by transvaginal laparoscopy vs standard laparoscopy is presented in Table 4.1. There were no difficulties in inspecting the cul-de-sac, the posterior wall of the uterus, or the uterosacral ligament using transvaginal laparoscopy. However, the tubes with all their parts, the ovaries and all its sides, and both fossae were evaluated in 87.0, 89.8, and 66.7% of the patients, respectively.

Table 4.1 Successful evaluation of the pelvis

Structure	Standard laparoscopy	Transvaginal laparoscopy
Pouch of Douglas (%)	100	100
Posterior wall of the uterus + sacrouterine ligament (%)	100	100
Tubes (%)	100	87
Ovaries (%)	100	89.8
Ovarian fossa (%)	100	66.7

Reproduced with permission from Darai et al.[4]

Another study[5] showed that patients with minimal and mild endometriosis and unexplained infertility had significantly more ovarian adhesions on transvaginal hydrolaparoscopy than on standard laparoscopy. The subtle adhesions seen on transvaginal hydrolaparoscopy but not on standard laparoscopy were filmy, microvascularized, and non-connecting.

A multicenter prospective study reported by Watrelot et al[6] comprising 81 patients, compared the two endoscopic techniques of laparoscopy and fertiloscopy in the routine evaluation of the pelvis in infertile women. The findings using the two endoscopic methods were strictly concordant in 65 patients (80%), among whom 47 patients showed morphologic abnormalities (positive/positive) and 16 had normal findings (negative/negative). There were 17 instances of discordant findings, either negative/positive in nine cases (11%) or positive/negative in eight cases (10%).

These results confirm that transvaginal laparoscopy is a minimally invasive and safe procedure that may be considered as an alternative to diagnostic laparoscopy in the routine assessment of women without clinical or ultrasonographic evidence of pelvic disease.

References

1. Gordts S, Campo R, Rombauts L, Brosens I. Endoscopic visualization of the process of fimbrial ovum retrieval in the human. Hum Reprod 1998; 13: 1425–8.
2. Puttemans P, Brosens I, Delattin P, Vasquez G, Boeckx W. Salpingoscopy versus hysterosalpingography in hydrosalpinges. Hum Reprod 1987; 2: 535–40.
3. Campo R, Gordts S, Rombauts L, Brosens I. Diagnostic accuracy of transvaginal hydrolaparoscopy in infertility. Fert Steril 1999; 71: 1157–60.
4. Darai E, Dessolle L, Lecuru F, Soriano D Transvaginal hydrolaparoscopy compared with laparoscopy for the evaluation of infertile women: a prospective comparative blind study. Hum Reprod 2000;15: 2379-82.
5. Brosens I, Gordts S, Campo R. Transvaginal hydrolaparoscopy but not standard laparoscopy reveals subtle endometriotic adhesions of the ovary. Fert Steril 2001; 75: 1009–12.
6. Watrelot A, Nisolle M, Chelli H et al. Is laparoscopy still the gold standard in infertility assessment? A comparison of fertiloscopy versus laparoscopy in infertility: Results of an international multicentre prospective trial: The 'FLY' (Fertiloscopy-LaparoscopY) study. Hum Reprod 2003; 18: 834–9.

5

Risks and complications of transvaginal access to the peritoneal cavity

Hugo Christian Verhoeven and Ivo Brosens

The fundamentals of peritoneal access in pelvic endoscopy have been extensively investigated in standard laparoscopy, but less for the transvaginal access. Reviews on complications in gynecologic laparoscopy reveal that risks and complications rates greatly vary, depending on the design of the survey (retrospective, prospective, or combined), type of survey (personal series, including learning period), extent of experience (reference centers, nationwide), type of laparoscopy (diagnostic, sterilization, operative), outcome measurements (type and degree of lesions, conversion to laparotomy), patients characteristics (body weight, predisposing factors) and type of anesthesia (local, general). Transvaginal access has been less investigated, but data are available on culdoscopy, insufflation through the cul-de-sac and, recently, on transvaginal hydrolaparoscopy. The risks and complications of these different techniques using the transvaginal access to the peritoneal cavity are reviewed.

Culdoscopy

The technique of culdoscopy was introduced in the early 1940s by Decker.[1] Culdoscopy allowed the endoscopic visualization of the pelvic organs through a transvaginal puncture into the cul-de-sac, with the patient in the knee-chest, or genupectoral, position. However, it was originally conceived as a complex hospital procedure with an uncomfortable and unstable position for the patient and an unusual orientation for the physician. The technology of sedating and anesthetizing the conscious patient was not as advanced then as now and presented problems of comfort for the patient and of control for the gynecologist. The advent of laparoscopy with the panoramic view of the pelvis was in the early 1960s seen as the answer to some of the problems and became the more popular method and achieved great popularity for its operative superiority. Today, laparoscopy has become largely an operative proce-

dure and is considered too invasive as a diagnostic procedure in patients without obvious pelvic pathology. However, the pioneers of pelvic endoscopy such as Raoul Palmer in Europe and Eduard Diamond in the USA appreciated culdoscopy as the method of choice for the diagnosis of infertility.

In 1978, Diamond[2] reported on a series of 4000 outpatient procedures over a period of 10 years in patients with infertility. For diagnostic purpose, he used the 8 mm, 90° Wolf endoscope through a 9 mm sleeve. The patient was to self-administer a Fleet enema the night before the culdoscopy appointment. A local anesthetic was applied and a pneumoperitoneum was created using initially air and later CO_2. Antibiotics were given routinely postoperatively for 7 days.

The complications of consecutive series are described in detail in Table 5.1. No death occcured in the entire series of culdoscopies. In six patients bleeding was prolonged, requiring suturing of the puncture site. Three patients developed pelvic peritonitis despite the routine use of antibiotics. One patient developed a pelvic abscess and was

Table 5.1 Complications in consecutive series of patients with infertility

	Complication (%)	
	Culdoscopy in 4000 patients[2]	TVL in 1000 patients[3]
Failed access	1	1.1
Major complication	0	0
Minor bleeding	0.15	2.3
Infection	0.07	0.2
Rectum perforation	0.12	0.5
Inadvert ovarian cyst puncture	0.1	0

TVL, transvaginal laparoscopy.

found to have unrecognized tuberculosis. Five inadvert trocar punctures into the rectum occurred, all of them during the first 5 years of the series and none during the later years. None of these patients required hospitalization or laparotomy and all were treated conservatively with antibiotics. Puncture of ovarian cysts that had prolapsed into the cul-de-sac occurred in four patients. No other complications associated with culdoscopy, such as perforation of intestines within the peritoneal cavity or perforation of an hydrosalpinx, occurred.

Contraindications included active pelvic inflammatory disease (PID), bleeding disorder, orthopedic deformity, a narrow vagina, and cul-de-sac obliterations. Diamond demonstrated that the feasibility, reliability, and safety of the procedure depended upon the skills of the culdoscopy team, which included training and experience, and, even more important, the selection of the appropriate candidates for culdoscopy. This was particularly evident from the extremely low morbidity and complication rates reported in his series. His conclusion in 1978 was that outpatient diagnostic culdoscopy should be returned to gynecologic training programs.

Cul-de-sac insufflation

Veress needle insertion through the cul-de-sac for insufflation has been used in difficult patients. With the patient in the Trendelenburg position, a single-tooth tenaculum is used to grasp and place the posterior cervix in anterior traction to tauten the posterior vaginal fornix. The tip of a long Veress needle is placed precisely in the midline, nearly 2 cm behind the junction of the rugae of the vaginal vault and the smooth epithelium of the cervical lip, and slowly advanced to no more than 3 cm.

Two series were published on the use of cul-de-sac insufflation for inducing pneumoperitoneum and they reported, respectively, a failure in 3.7% for a series of 107 women[4] and 2.1% for a series of 570 patients.[5] No complications were reported.

Transvaginal hydrolaparoscopy

The specific features of transvaginal laparoscopy (TVL), in contrast to culdoscopy as described by Diamond, are that the patient lies in the dorsal decubitus position and that prewarmed saline or buffered saline or Ringer's lactate is used for the distention of the peritoneal cavity.[6] A small-diameter (<3.5 mm), foroblique 30°, wide-angled and rigid optic is used. Inspection of the pelvic structures is achieved without grasping or manipulation. At the end of the procedure, a chromopertubation test is performed and, when

indicated, salpingoscopy is added. All interventions at our center are performed under conscious sedation as an office procedure in an outpatient surgical suite.

TVL is considered complete if the tubo-ovarian structures, pelvic sidewalls, and cul-de-sac can be seen, or if pathology is diagnosed that indicates the need for operative intervention or assisted reproductive technology (ART).

Complications

We reported recently on our personal (HV, first author) series of 1000 consecutive TVL procedures that were performed during the period from 1998 until 2003.[3] Access with good visualization was obtained in 96.8% of the patients. Unexpected major pathology was diagnosed in 232 patients (24%) and included mainly ovarian endometriosis, tubo-ovarian adhesions, isthmic block, and hydrosalpinges. The diagnostic findings resulted in 36 (3.7%) operative laparoscopies and 204 (21.1%) medical therapies and ARTs.

No major complications occurred in this series. The main complications were intraperitoneal bleeding and rectum perforation. Intraperitoneal bleeding was seen in 23 (2.3%) of the patients and occurred on the posterior wall of the uterus ($n = 13$), parametrium ($n = 2$), ovary ($n = 2$), omentum ($n = 1$), and adhesions ($n = 3$). Rectum perforation occurred in five patients (0.5%) and was managed conservatively with antibiotics. Infection occurred in two patients (0.2%) (see Table 5.1).

Selection of patients

Transvaginal endoscopy, including mini-hysteroscopy and transvaginal hydrolaparoscopy, has been proposed as a first-line endoscopy-based infertility investigation to evaluate the uterine cavity, tubal patency, and normality of the tubo-ovarian structures in patients with no obvious or major cause of infertility. The technique is intended to replace and improve the findings which are currently evaluated by hysterosalpingography, in particular the uterine cavity, tubal patency, and the normality of the tubo-ovarian structures. Therefore, the main indication is the investigation of infertile patients without obvious pelvic pathology.

The contraindications include the presence of lower genital tract infection, active PID, a cul-de-sac obstruction, and the presence of a prolapsed ovarian tumor in the cul-de-sac. It is therefore most important to select the patient carefully by history, gynecologic examination, and vaginal sonography. The prevention of complications is summarized in Table 5.2.

Table 5.2 Prevention of complications

History and gynecological examination to exclude:
- genital tract infection
- fixed retroverted or laterally deviated uterus
- retrocervical or rectovaginal endometriosis
- cul-de-sac obliteration

Transvaginal sonography to exclude:
- large ovarian cyst
- cul-de-sac tumor

Limit the number of attempts to enter the peritoneal cavity to three

Avoid sweeping movements with the Veress needle

Verify the intraperitoneal position of the needle

Antibiotics and close follow-up in the event of rectal perforation, risk of flare-up of pelvic inflammatory disease, or inadvert puncture of an ovarian endometrioma

Failed identification of pelvic structures

Visualization during TVL can be obscured by the presence of bleeding. Bleeding from the insertion site or from inadvert needle puncture of the posterior side of the uterus or other site may be a problem in the early stages, but in experienced hands bleeding is rarely a cause of failure of inspection.

In the absence of a panoramic view, the pelvic structures are identified by moving back and forward and rotating the optic along the tissues. The full inspection of the pelvic structures needs to be performed in a systematic way and is therefore more time consuming than at laparoscopy. However, it is essential to master the technique before taking on even minor surgical procedures.

Chiesa-Montadou et al[7] recently reported two complications occurring during ovarlan capsule drilling using the fertiloscope. In the first case, the insertion of a bipolar electrode into the ovary to a depth of about 0.5 mm caused bleeding from the ovarian stroma which could not be controlled and required conversion to laparoscopy. In the second case, an intestinal loop was taken for the ovary and only after several punctures and coagulations the error became obvious. Both cases occurred before 50 cases of diagnostic fertiloscopy had been performed.

Rectum perforation

The potentially serious complication of transvaginal needle access is rectal perforation and sepsis. In a multinational survey comprising 3667 procedures by either transvaginal hydrolaparoscopy or fertiloscopy the incidence of bowel perforation was 0.65%, which decreased after initial experience to 0.25%.[8] No delayed diagnosis or sepsis occurred and all except one case were managed with outpatient antibiotics. Laparotomy was performed in one case where a surgeon consultant recommended an explorative laparotomy.

We confirmed, as previously observed by Diamond,[2] that a small needle perforation of the rectum can be managed conservatively by outpatient observation and antibiotics. It is interesting to note that Diamond reported a very low rate of rectum perforations by the trocar. The difference can be explained by several factors, including the genupectoral position or the technique of achieving access to the peritoneal cavity. Bowel injuries caused by a Veress needle are likely to be less severe than those produced by a trocar and therefore they are also likely to be underreported. In transvaginal hydrolaparoscopy, a Veress needle–trocar system is used and the insertion site of the Veress needle is controlled by introducing the optic through the Veress needle sleeve to inspect the position of the Veress needle. In Diamond's series, the trocar was inserted separately after Veress needle insertion and the creation of a pneumoperitoneum.

In general, bowel injuries caused by the insertion of the trocar require surgical repair, whereas Veress needle injuries are apparently managed conservatively. In a Dutch survey,[9] three cases of stomach injury by Veress needle were diagnosed and treated expectantly without adverse outcome. In a multinational survey, Brosens and Gordon[10,11] reported that Veress needle bowel injury was treated expectantly in four cases and by laparotomy and simple closure in three other cases. One case of a tear and fistula of 12 mm was reported, indicating that sweeping movements with a Veress needle at the time of perforation can cause a major bowel injury that requires surgical repair.

The majority of bowel injuries caused during transvaginal hydrolaporoscopy involve the retroperitoneal rectum with healthy bowel tissue. Usually the injury is small, measuring between 2 and 6 mm, and shows no leakage. Therefore, the injury caused under standard conditions at the time of insertion of the small-diameter endoscopic system can be considered as a minor lesion. The most detrimental factor in bowel complication is the delay of the diagnosis of a bowel injury. Therefore, a system that allows the diagnosis of the perforation at the time of insertion may yield a higher incidence, but at the same time may decrease the risk of delayed diagnosis and severe complications of a bowel injury.

Learning curve

Analysis of the occurrence of complications in relation to experience confirms the importance of the learning period.

The correlation of the failures (no access or no visualization) with the experience showed that five (10%) failures occurred in the first 50 procedures, and 26 (2.8%) in the subsequent 950 procedures ($p = 0.028$). Bleeding occurred in 5 (10%) of the first 50 cases and in 18 (1.9%) of the following 950 cases ($p = 0.004$). Rectum perforation occurred in four (8%) of the first 50 cases and in one (0.1%) of the following 950 cases ($p<0.0001$). In total, after the initial 50 cases, the complication rate of intraperitoneal bleeding and bowel perforation decreased in our personal series significantly respectively, from 1.9% to 0.1%.

A similar decrease of rectum perforations in relation to experience was a significant finding in the multinational survey on transvaginal access using the TVL and fertiloscope techniques.[8] After the initial experience of 50 cases, the prevalence of bowel injury was 0.25%. All the injuries were diagnosed during the procedure and no delayed diagnosis occurred. In addition, 22 (92%) cases were managed conservatively without consequences.

Finally, the publication of two complications during operative fertiloscopy underlines that there is a learning curve which appears to require a minimum of 50 cases.

Conclusions

In conclusion, the available data confirm that transvaginal hydrolaparoscopy is a safe technique for pelvic inspection and tubal patency testing in patients with infertility. However, the technique requires a training and a learning period. It should be stressed that complications can occur even in experienced hands. In addition to the skills and experience required, the most important aspect for the prevention of complications is the selection of patients.

References

1. Decker A. Culdoscopy – A New Technique in Gynecology and Obstetric Diagnosis. Philadelphia: WB Saunders, 1952.
2. Diamond E. Diagnostic culdoscopy in infertility: a study of 4,000 outpatient procedures. J Reprod Med 1978; 21: 23–30.
3. Verhoeven H, Gordts S, Campo R, Brosens I. Role of transvaginal hydrolaparoscopy in the investigation of female infertility: a review of 1000 procedures. Gynecol Surg 2004; 1: 191–3.
4. Neely MR, McWilliams R, Makhlouf HA. Laparoscopy: routine pneumoperitoneum via the posterior fornix. Obstet Gynecol 1975; 45: 459–60.
5. van Schie KJ, van Lith DA, Beekhuizen W, du Plessis-Alblas M. Cul-de-sac insufflation to induce pneumoperitoneum: an analysis of rare problems. Int J Gynaecol Obstet 1980; 18: 245–7.
6. Gordts S, Campo R, Rombauts L, Brosens I. Transvaginal hydrolaparoscopy as an outpatient procedure for infertility investigation. Hum Reprod 1998; 13: 99–103.
7. Chiesa-Montadou S, Rongieres C, Garbin O, Nisand I. About two complications of ovarian drilling by fertiloscopy. Gynecol Obstet Fertil 2003; 31: 844–6 [in French].
8. Gordts S, Watrelot A, Campo R et al. Risk and outcome of bowel injury during transvaginal pelvic endoscopy. Fertil Steril 2001, 76: 1238–41.
9. Jansen FW, Kapiteyn K, Trimbos-Kemper T et al. Complications of laparoscopy: a prospective multicentre observational study. Br J Obstet Gynaecol 1997; 104: 595–600.
10. Brosens I, Gordon A. Bowel injuries during gynaecological laparoscopy. Gynaecol Endosc 2001; 10: 141–5.
11. Brosens I, Gordon A, Campo R, Gordts S. Bowel injury in gynecologic laparoscopy. J Am Assoc Gynecol Laparosc 2003; 10: 9–13.

Section II

Pathology at transvaginal endoscopy

6

Fertility-enhancing hysteroscopic surgery

Yves Van Belle and Patrick Puttemans

Introduction

In this chapter the indications, possibilities, and techniques of operative hysteroscopy in the infertile patient are described. This also means that the ablation of the endometrium, e.g. for menstrual disorders in premenopausal women, will not be covered here.

When we compare the findings in a symptomatic gynecological population and a screening program in an infertile patient group, it is striking that the screening procedure detects as much pathology as the symptomatic population. Those findings support the idea that it is absolutely necessary to perform an ambulatory diagnostic hysteroscopy in every infertile patient. Moreover, when we compare the pathologies found in a standard gynecological population with those of infertile patients, we see that the infertile population group is characterized by a higher incidence of congenital pathology and a lower incidence of acquired pathology. Those findings confirm that it is absolutely necessary to perform an office hysteroscopy also in every in vitro fertilization (IVF) or intracytoplasmic sperm injection (ICSI) candidate. The advantages of mini-hysteroscopy have been demonstrated prospectively and significantly as a first-line diagnostic tool in an office setting[1] and this mini-hysteroscopy is now used in

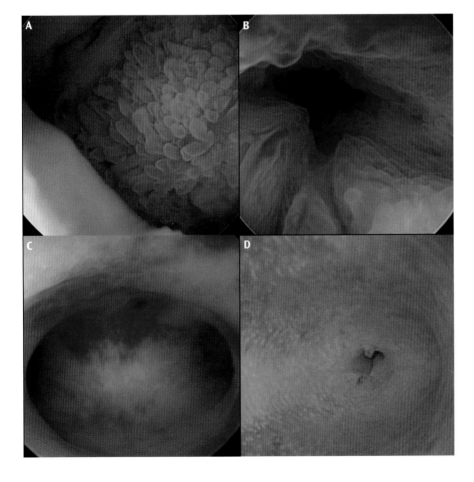

Figure 6.1
Normal images of (a) exocervix, (b) endocervical canal, (c) uterine cavity, and (d) tubal ostium as seen during an office mini-hysteroscopy.

the department on a daily basis (Figure 6.1) without the use of a speculum or a tenaculum and with saline, at body temperature and 100 mmHg, as a distension medium.

Magnetic resonance imaging (MRI) has revealed that the endometrio–myometrial interface constitutes a distinct, hormone-dependent uterine compartment called the junctional zone. In the non-pregnant uterus, highly specialized contraction waves originate exclusively from the junctional zone and participate in the regulation of diverse reproductive events, such as sperm transport, embryo implantation, and menstrual shedding. Conversely, growing evidence suggests that disruption of the normal endometrio–myometrial interface plays an integral role in diverse reproductive disorders.[2] Besides the well-known example of adenomyosis, fibroids may or may not originate from that junctional zone. It means that these 'junctional zone myomas' (i.e. most submucous and some intramural fibroids) may well interfere with embryo implantation and development. And that is where, in our opinion, hysteroscopic surgery will become even more important than it already is today: by the safe removal, not only of type 0 and type 1 submucous fibroids but also of type 2 submucous and of some intramural fibroids, provided there is a safety margin between the fibroid and the uterine serosa, with the use of bipolar cutting power via specially adapted loop electrodes in a harmless distension medium without the risk of fluid overload and toxicity.

Congenital pathology and infertility

Prevalence

> The incidence of congenital uterine anomalies is difficult to establish, because not all anomalies induce symptoms or are related to infertility.

In the literature we find a great variation in incidence, from 0.2% up to 10%. This variation is probably due to the different populations studied and because of the frequent subjective interpretation of the different findings. The prospective registration of pathologic findings during mini-hysteroscopy in Leuven between 1993 and 1995 (Table 6.1),[3] comparing a normal population to a group of infertile patients, indicated a significantly higher incidence of congenital anomalies in the infertile population (13.2%) in comparison to the standard population (1.7%).

Acién[4] found an overall incidence of Müllerian defects in 7–8% of the general population and in >25% of women with a history of recurrent miscarriage. However, clear uterine malformations are observed in 5% of the general

Table 6.1 Prevalence of congenital uterine malformations

Congenital malformations prevalence	N	%
Total examinations	530	100
Normal findings	370	69.8
Abnormal findings:	151	28.5
• congenital	70	13.2
• acquired	21	3.9
• subtle	60	11.3
No diagnosis	9	1.7
Congenital anomalies	70	100
• uterine septum	44	63
• uterus infantilis	16	23
• 'T-shaped' uterus	7	10
• uterus unicornis	3	4

population, in 2–3% of the fertile women, in 3% of infertile patients, in 5–10% of patients with recurrent miscarriage, and in >25% of the patients with both late abortions and immature deliveries.

Detailed analysis of the different anomalies found in the infertile population indicates the important role of a uterine septum in the infertile patient. Appropriate diagnosis by hysteroscopy, if necessary in combination with laparoscopy, echography, hydrosonography (Figure 6.2), and MRI, and extrapolating these findings to the obstetrical history of the patient, demonstrates that neither the bicornuate nor the dydelphic nor the unicornuate uterus plays an important role in infertility.

The infantile uterus is characterized by a normal formed cavum but the corpus/cervix relation is the same as in the juvenile uterus, namely ⅓. Infertility in those cases is more a result of the accompanying ovarian insufficiency than of an aberrantly formed organ.

The 'T-shaped' uterus is usually a very rare finding but due to the intake of diethylstilbestrol by approx. 2–3 million pregnant women between 1941 and 1971, its influence will last until the year 2010.

Classification

Mainly as a result of the different diagnostic and therapeutic modalities over the years, it has been difficult to obtain a detailed anatomical description of the anomaly in an easy manner. This has led to different and sometimes very confusing classifications.

Modern diagnostic modalities such as office mini-hysteroscopy, ultrasound, contrast ultrasound, MRI, and laparoscopy enable us to gather detailed anatomical

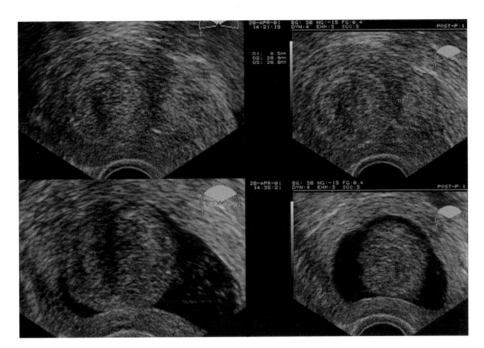

Figure 6.2
Added value of transvaginal
ultrasound (top row) and
hydrosonography (bottom row),
here in the case of a type 0
submucous myoma.

descriptions in a simple, safe, and efficient way. The introduction of hysteroscopic treatment modalities for several
anomalies has dramatically changed the invasiveness of the
intervention. Taking into account these changed diagnostic
and operative modalities, we believe that the American Fertility Society classification[5] should be modified according
to the pathogenesis and the possibility or necessity of a
minimally invasive surgical correction.

Congenital malformations class 1 and 2

- Class 1: bilateral total or partial agenesis or hypoplasia
  of the Müllerian ducts.
- Class 2: uterus unicornis with or without a rudimentary, contralateral horn (Figure 6.3).

These anomalies have the same pathogenic origin: class 1
reflects bilateral and class 2 unilateral total or partial agenesis or hypoplasia of the Müllerian ducts.

A typical example of class 1 anomaly is the Mayer–Roki-
tansky–Küster–Hauser syndrome in which the patient is
sterile and pregnancy can only occur with the help of sur-
rogate parenting.

Class 2 anomalies will present themselves at hysteroscopy as a single uterine horn; yet other examinations
are needed to determine the presence and/or the activity of
a contralateral horn. A non-communicating contralateral
horn with active, i.e. hormone-dependent, endometrium
will manifest its presence in normal menstruating adoles-
cents (14–16 years old) complaining of a painful pelvic
mass and severe dysmenorrhea.

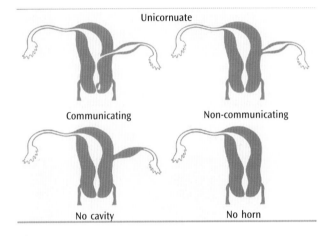

Unicornuate

Communicating   Non-communicating

No cavity   No horn

Figure 6.3
Uterus uncornis with or without a rudimentary, contralateral
horn.

Congenital malformations class 3

- Class 3: uterus didelphys and uterus unicollis bicornis
  (bicornuate uterus) (Figures 6.4 and 6.5).

Here the anomaly originates from incomplete or absence
of fusion of the ductus paramesonephrici, resulting in different degrees of horn formation. Vaginal and urinary tract
anomalies frequently accompany this malformation. Both
anomalies have similar diagnostic features, comparable
influence on pregnancy outcome and, if surgery is indicated, the same procedure needs to be followed.

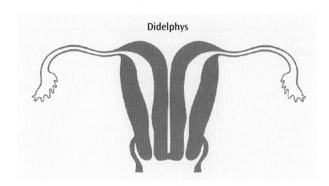

Figure 6.4
Uterus didelphys.

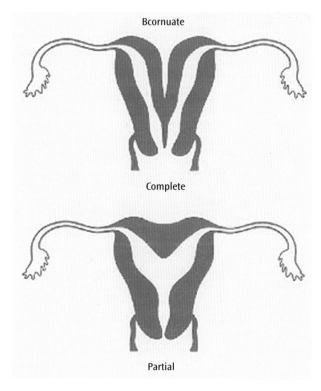

Figure 6.5
Uterus unicollis bicornis.

Diagnosis can only be established by combined examinations. Once the midline fundal uterine muscle is larger than 15 mm, we define the malformation as being a mixture between a bicornuate and a septated uterus.

Congenital malformations class 4

• Class 4: uterus septus and uterus subseptus (Figure 6.6).

These anomalies are due to the insufficient resorption of the sagittal uterine wall.

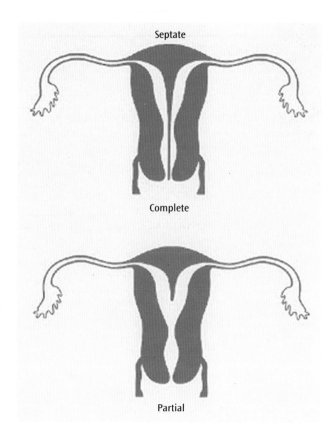

Figure 6.6
Uterus septus and subseptus.

The outline of the uterus is perfectly normal and there is no sign of horn formation at ultrasound, MRI, or laparoscopy. A lot of publications indicate that the septate uterus can be a cause of recurrent abortions. The possible reason for frequent early abortions is seen as the fact that the blastocyst often implants on the lower part of the septum. Contrary to the normal uterine wall, here we find a different and less-developed vascular architecture that could be responsible for a disturbed nidation or placentation. If and why nidation occurs preferably on the septum is unknown. It has been reported that the evolution of a pregnancy can be without any problems, despite the presence of a uterine septum.

Congenital malformations class 5

• Class 5: T-shaped uterine cavity (Figure 6.7).

The typical T shape is best seen on a hysterosalpingogram. At hysteroscopy we see a narrow cavity with a cylindrical shape, whereas in the fundal region the uterine horns and the tubal ostia can only be visualized by lateral rotation of the 30° optic. The fundal thickness measured with ultrasound should be between 9 and 13 mm and is never thicker than 15 mm.

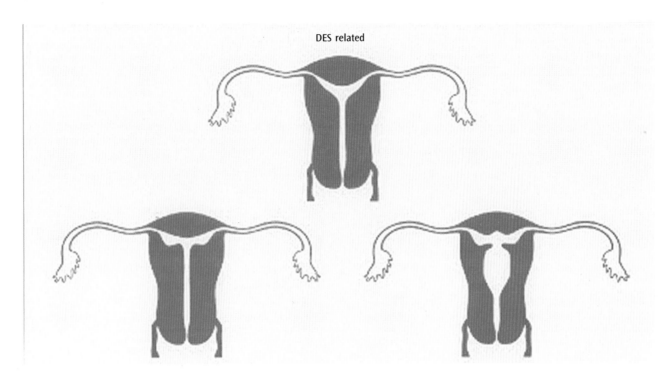

DES related

Figure 6.7
T-shaped uterine cavity.

In different detailed studies, Kaufman et al[6–8] analyzed the reproductive outcome of diethylstilbestrol (DES)-exposed patients with and without deformations of the uterine cavity at hysterosalpingography. These results did not justify an abdominal metroplasty for a T-shaped uterus. With the introduction of small-sized operative hysteroscopes and appropriate electrosurgical generators and electrodes however, the hysteroscopic reconstruction of the T shape into a normal triangular cavity can be achieved quite easily.

Congenital malformations class 6

Class 6 are those anomalies like infantile, hypoplastic, or arcuate uterus (Figure 6.8), which are variations on the normal pear-like shape of the uterine cavity but where no surgical correction can be made. The infantile uterus is characterized by a normally formed cavum but the corpus/cervix relation is the same as in the juvenile uterus, namely ⅓.

What is being discussed is that infertility in those cases is more a result of the accompanying ovarian insufficiency rather than due to an aberrantly formed organ.

Congenital malformations class 7

These are those rare anomalies that cannot be classified correctly in any of the above-mentioned classes.

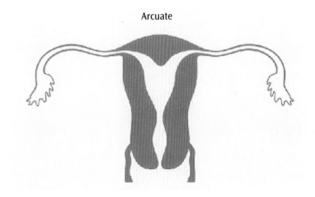

Arcuate

Figure 6.8
Arcuate uterus.

Acquired pathology and infertility

Prevalence

Deformation of the uterine cavity due to important acquired pathology like an intrauterine myoma, large (>1 cm) endometrial polyps, and partial or total cavity occlusion is less frequent in infertile patients than in the normal population. Fibroids or endometrial polyps inside the uterine cavity are often suspected at vaginal ultrasound, i.e. before the office mini-hysteroscopy.

Table 6.2 Hysteroscopic classification of submucous myomas

Type 0	the complete circumference of this myoma lies within the uterine cavity
Type I	more than 50% of the fibroid's diameter lies within the uterine cavity
Type II	less than 50% of the fibroid's diameter lies within the lining of the uterine cavity

Classification

Polyps

The importance of gynecological polyps in general and of endocervical, endometrial or tubal polyps in particular is unclear. Prospective scientific data are lacking, but on the other hand most gynecologists tend to remove large endometrial polyps systematically. They are a cause of abnormal uterine bleeding, most often not related to the patient's cycle, and the fact that these polyps may grow and/or bleed during the first trimester of a pregnancy, i.e. alarming both the patient and her physician, is the main reason for their systematic removal. The polyp itself or its bleeding may well interfere with embryo implantation. In young patients it is rare to remove these polyps for oncological reasons, but with the advancing age of the infertile patient, one needs to take into account the possibility of hyperplasia or even endometrial cancer within the polyp, or, for instance, a metastasis from a breast cancer. And therefore the removal of a polyp offers another advantage, namely a detailed histological diagnosis. The role, if any, of tiny endocervical polyps, or of very small polyps near or inside the tubal ostium is unclear. Although these very small polyps are a frequent finding at hysteroscopy, most fertility specialists are reluctant to use electrocautery within the endocervical canal or the tubal ostium, since that procedure itself may induce postoperative stenosis. Polyps of less then 1 mm are usually left in place. The others can be removed using microscissors.

Myoma

Uterine fibroids can be found frequently. Depending on their anatomical localization, we divide them into submucous, intramural, and subserous myoma.

Their significance for fertility is not very clear. It is possible that intracavitary myoma interfere with reproduction in the same way as an intrauterine device does. Histologic studies have shown that intramural and submucous myoma can alternate and change the endometrial and myometrial structure. Subserous fibroids probably do not influence fertility and mostly represent an asymptomatic finding. Hysteroscopy plays an important role in determining what type of myoma is present (Table 6.2) and whether surgery on a myoma is indicated or required. Both the intracavitary localization and the reactive hypervascularization seen at hysteroscopy are arguments in favor of the influence the myoma might have on the endometrium. The same is probably true for some of the intramural fibroids that originate in the junctional zone.

Synechiae

Intrauterine adhesions or synechiae occur mostly in women with a problem of secondary infertility. The cause can be a post-traumatic, post-infectious, or postoperative adhesion formation, e.g. after a dilatation and curettage (D&C) for miscarriage, cesarean section, or intrauterine surgery with diathermy. In the vast majority of cases, intrauterine adhesions are caused by intrauterine instrumental manipulations in relation to a pregnancy. Adhesion formation not related to an obstetric intervention is quite unusual but it may occur following intrauterine surgery, such as metroplasty, myomectomy, or D&C.

In cases of total obliteration and amenorrhea, it is not difficult to understand secondary infertility. In situations where there is only partial obliteration, it is unclear if an infertile situation exists because of reduction of the functional endometrial surface or because of disturbance of the endometrial vascularization.

Placental retention following a birth or miscarriage can also cause partial obliteration of the uterine cavity since it induces fibrin deposition and is a cause of both acute and chronic endometritis surrounding these tissue fragments. Vaginal ultrasound may already give an indication, but hysteroscopy is the gold standard for a correct diagnosis.

Subtle endometrial changes

Besides the diagnosis of major pathology such as uterine septa, polyps, myoma, synechia, or total cavity obliteration, mini-hysteroscopy, with the use of a watery distention medium, frequently indicates the presence of minimal or subtle changes of the endometrium. Moderate or marked mucosal elevations are possibly a sign for inappropriate hormonal stimulation of the endometrium.

Aberration of the vascular architecture of the endometrium is another lesion that could be important for reproductive performance and which can only be visualized by hysteroscopy.

Hypervascularization is often seen in the presence of a large intrauterine or intramural myoma but can also be seen as a solitary finding. In their series, Campo et al[3] found nine cases of endometrial hypervascularization, defined as a significantly increased amount of vessels in the proliferative phase or a reddish endometrium in which the white openings of the glands produce the typical strawberry-like pattern. Neither microbiology nor histology seems to have any diagnostic value in these cases. Only in one case was it possible to demonstrate the presence of a chronic endometritis histology. Cervical swabs showed the presence of *Gardnerella vaginalis* in two cases, *Escherichia coli* in one case, and streptococci group D infection in another patient. It was observed that in those nine cases, the hysteroscopic view normalized after 2 months of hormone replacement treatment combined with 10 days of antibiotic treatment. In two women with a problem of secondary infertility and where the hypervascularization was the only feature found, pregnancy occurred spontaneously within 6 months of drug treatment.

Mini-hysteroscopy plays a key role in the evaluation of different treatment modalities to restore the normal endometrial environment.

Operative hysteroscopy

Congenital pathology

Septum

Detailed analysis of the different anomalies found in the infertile population shows the important role of a uterine

Table 6.3 Uterine septum – pre- and postoperative reproductive outcome

	Preoperative		Postoperative	
	N	%	N	%
Total patients	43	100	31	100
Patients with 1 living child	10[a]	23.2	29*	93.5
Pregnancies:	117	100	37	100
• abortions	104[a]	88.9	5[a]	13.5
• premature	6	5.1	5	13.5
• at term	7	6.0	27	73
• live children	12[a]	10.2	32[a]	86.5

[a]$p < 0.001$

septum in the infertile patient.[9] Hysteroscopic surgery can be performed either with microscissors or with the bipolar needle (Figures 6.9 and 6.10). The flow of saline can be stopped whenever necessary to evaluate the presence of bleeding vessels, indicating that the incision of the septum is nearly complete. A second-look hysteroscopy is performed 8–10 weeks later, to rule out the presence of postoperative synechiae.

Table 6.3 shows the pre- and postoperative reproductive outcome of 61 consecutive infertile patients with the presence of an intrauterine septum. A partial septum was present in 51 cases, and a total septum was present in 10 cases.

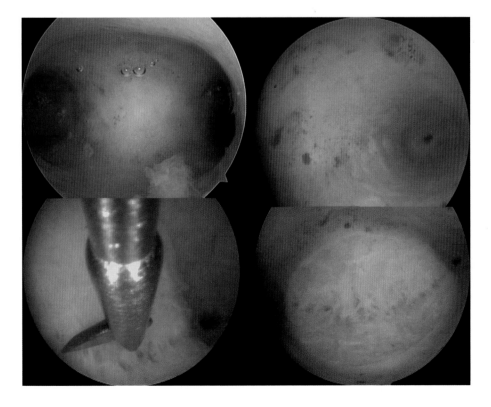

Figure 6.9
Four stages of the incision of a small septum (uterus subseptus) with the microscissors.

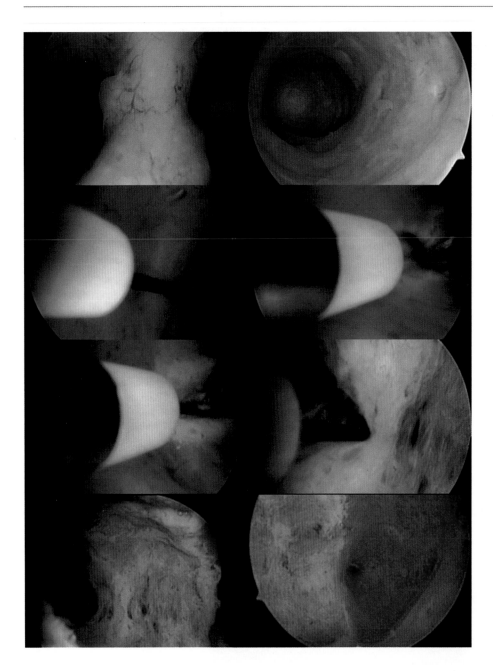

Figure 6.10
Eight stages of the incision of a big septum (uterus septus) with the bipolar needle.

Eighteen patients were suffering from primary infertility and the remaining 43 patients consulted with a problem of secondary infertility. Table 6.4 summarizes the above section on the uterine septum.

The reproductive performance of those 43 patients was very striking. In total, 117 pregnancies were recorded, 104 (88.9%) of which ended in an abortion. With the exception of one, all abortions were early ones. The 13 remaining pregnancies resulted in six preterm deliveries (one baby died) and in seven term deliveries only.

At the time of diagnosis of the septum, only 10 out of 43 patients had at least one living child. Comparing the incidence of abortions and the pregnancy outcome pre- and postoperatively there was a statistically significant decrease

in the abortion rate and a significant increase in the live birth rate and in uncomplicated pregnancies.

The 37 pregnancies listed represent 32 live births, five of which occurred before 36 weeks of gestation. In five patients an early abortion was diagnosed. One patient who had an ectopic pregnancy was not included in the statistics.

Of the 41 patients with secondary infertility, only 10 patients already had a living child. Postoperatively, 31 patients conceived, resulting in 29 patients with at least one living child. The results of hysteroscopic metroplasty are equal to those of transabdominal metroplasty. Hysteroscopic metroplasty in the patient's history is not an indication for an elective primary cesarean section: the delivery management can be the same as in a non-operated patient.

Table 6.4 Uterine septum – summary

- Uterus subseptus (partial septum) and septus (total septum) are the most frequent congenital uterine anomalies caused by an incomplete resorption of the Müllerian ducts
- Biostatistical analysis indicates that patients with a septate uterus have the worst reproductive outcome, with a high incidence of early miscarriages
- The hysteroscopic septum dissection has replaced the transabdominal metroplasty and is a relatively simple, safe, and, above all, efficient operative procedure, since it significantly increases the live birth rate in patients with recurrent pregnancy loss
- Not every patient with a septate uterus suffers from recurrent pregnancy loss, but these women present with a higher incidence of fetal malposition and Cesarean section
- The hysteroscopic septum dissection must be performed before starting an infertility treatment
- This endoscopic septum dissection does not improve the pregnancy rates in infertile patients

One should be aware of some case reports of uterine rupture after septum dissection and, in case of a remaining cervical septum, it may be necessary to remove it during vaginal delivery, since at full cervical dilation it may block the passage of the fetus. In the postpartal period, special attention should be given to the delivery of the placenta, because it is reported that there is a tendency towards a higher incidence of placenta acreta.

T-shaped cavity

The importance of the T-shaped uterine cavity for the patient's reproductive performance is not so clear as with the uterine septum. It seems, however, that patients with a T-shaped uterus are at higher risk for ectopic pregnancies and that the live birth rate is significantly lower than in normal fertile patients. In case of a T-shaped uterus, surgery aims to increase the size and to reconstruct the normal shape of the uterine cavity. The correction of a T-shaped cavity is technically more difficult than the incision of a septum, since one needs to carefully assess the location of both tubal ostia, the imaginary lines between both of them, and the imaginary lines from the isthmic part of the uterine cavity towards each ostium. This means one needs to make extensive use of the rotation of the 30° angle of the hysteroscope, in order to ensure the incision of both lateral walls with the bipolar needle in the correct plane. The total instrument diameter is also important, because the extremely small environment does not permit a cervical dilation until Hegar probe # 9 or 10. Microscissors can also

be used, but there is, for example, no room for a resectoscope. The VersaPoint needle is in our opinion way too powerful to make these tiny incisions. Moreover, the uterine artery and ureter are positioned in the lower lateral cervicouterine transition zone, i.e. the isthmical region of the uterus, and with the sideways incision of the uterine wall, we have no accessory tool to measure the depth of incision. In experienced hands, the hysteroscopic sidewall incision gives an excellent result from an anatomical point of view. From the patient's point of view, it is a relatively minor intervention in day care, with only minor discomfort. Both laparoscopy and ultrasound have no added value in these circumstances. The postoperative policy is the same as in the case of a uterine septum dissection: antibiotic prophylaxis, 2 months of sequential estrogen and progesterone administration, followed by an outpatient second-look hysteroscopy to evaluate the result and rule out the presence of postoperative intrauterine synechiae.

> There is only limited experience with this procedure, so definite conclusions regarding reproductive outcome cannot be made. The first results of small studies indicate an improvement of the term pregnancy rate but no change of the implantation rate.

Other congenital anomalies, such as a uterus didelphys or bicornuate uterus, do not necessitate endoscopic surgery.

Anomalies with hematometra

> In very rare instances we can find an anomaly in which a cavity with functional endometrium is not connected with the cervix and vagina combined with a contralateral cavity with normal access to the cervix and vagina. This situation can originate from a total septum where the lower part of the septum closes one cavity or from a bicornual uterus with one rudimentary horn. This combination of hematometra with normal menstruation can be challenging to diagnose. One should be aware of those situations when a painful abdominal mass is found in the normally menstruating adolescent, especially when there is a relationship between the pain and the menstrual cycle.

The clinical picture for both situations is typical: in the case of a uterine septum with one non-communicating cavity, we find at the menarche first a secondary dysmenorrhea, which increases in the following menstrual cycles. As a result of menstrual reflux, endometriosis will be generated and, progressively, a hematometra will occur in the occluded cavity. Frequently, the diagnosis is missed because of its rare occurrence, difficult recognition at

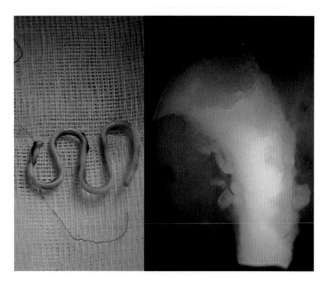

Figure 6.11
From the department 'lost and found': unexplained infertility in a young Cuban couple, unaware of the IUD (Lippes loop, that is difficult to see on ultrasound since it doesn't contain copper) that must have been inserted in their native country following an abortion many years ago; the scheduled IVF was cancelled and the patient became pregnant 3 months later.

laparoscopy, and frequent correlation with severe endometriosis, which is held responsible for the pain history. Only by performing a hysteroscopy can one observe the unicorn aspect of the cavity by normal laparoscopic uterine appearance. Modern vaginal sonography will certainly contribute to make a fast and accurate diagnosis.

In the case of a unicorn uterus with functional non-communicating rudimentary horn, supplementary to the above-mentioned symptoms, the presence of an abdominal mass will occur.

The treatment of a complete and occluding septum is the same as that already described. The difficulty here is to find a way to the occluded cavity. With the use of the cutting needle on the midline, and under (abdominal) ultrasound guidance, a passage is found. Entering the occluded cavity, old blood and mucus will blur the vision. Once visualization is restored, the opening is enlarged as much as possible. In the case of a very small cavity, it can be advisable to perform a cutting loop ablation to prevent recurrence of the hematometra. In this way, a hemiuterus extirpation or hysterectomy can be avoided.

In the case of a rudimentary contralateral horn, we recommend the removal of this horn by laparoscopy or laparotomy. In the case of a hysteroscopic approach, the objective is to find a passage to the contralateral horn and to perform an ablative destruction of the endometrium.

Acquired pathology

Placental retention, lost intrauterine device

This pathology (Figures 6.11 and 6.12) can be dealt with using mechanical operative hysteroscopy without the use whatsoever of electrical current and with the use of antibiotics preoperatively. The risk that the accompanying endometritis is inducing synechiae is indeed too high.

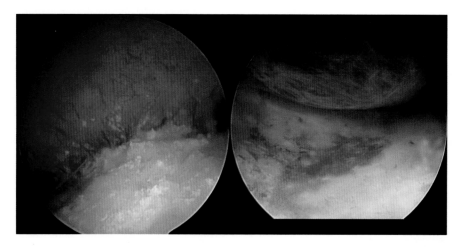

Figure 6.12
Two examples of remaining placental fragments including fibrosis and severe endometritis following a delivery, miscarriage, or D&C for miscarriage or abortion. The treatment consists of an operative hysteroscopy with the loop electrode, which is only used in a mechanical way, i.e. without any form of electrical current, to separate these tissue fragments from the endometrial layer. Antibiotics, Methergin (methylergonorine maleate), and a second-look hysteroscopy 8–10 weeks later are strongly indicated to avoid and rule out postoperative synechiae.

Grade	Extent of IUA
Table 6.5 Classification of IUAs (intrauterine adhesions) according to K Wamsteker and ESGE*	
I	Thin and/or filmy adhesions: • easily ruptured with the hysteroscope itself • corneal
II	A single dense adhesion: • connecting separate areas of the uterine cavity • visualization of both tubal ostia is possible • the adhesion cannot be ruptured by the hysteroscope alone
IIa	Occluding adhesions only in the region of the internal cervical os: • whereas the upper part of the uterine cavity is normal
III	Multiple dense adhesions: • connecting separate areas of the uterine cavity • unilateral obliteration of the ostial areas of the Fallopian tubes (see Figure 6.13)
IV	Extensive dense adhesions with (partial) occlusion of the uterine cavity: • and with both tubal ostial areas (partially) occluded
Va	Extensive endometrial scarring and fibrosis in combination with grade I or grade II adhesions: • with amenorrhea or pronounced hypo(spanio)menorrhea
Vb	Extensive endometrial scarring and fibrosis in combination with grade III or grade IV adhesions • with amenorrhea

*European Society for Gynecological Oncology (www.esge.org).

Synechiae

Lysis of endocervical or intrauterine adhesions can only be performed with the hysteroscope if the adhesions are very thin and fragile. In all other cases, the adhesions should be cut with 'micro'scissors under direct visual control. Pushing with the hysteroscope against adhesions to try to rupture them is too traumatic, can be the cause of recurrences and can easily lead to perforation of the uterine wall.

Minor intrauterine adhesions (grades I, II and Va) (Table 6.5; Figure 6.13) can be treated immediately during a diagnostic ambulant hysteroscopy. The use of local anesthesia is preferred in grade II adhesions as an operative hysteroscope is required. The adhesions can be cut with either type of hysteroscopic endosurgery: conventional scissors, Nd:YAG laser, or resection with a mono- or bipolar needle. However, as the uterine cavity is generally somewhat narrowed in case of intrauterine synechiae, even the use of a small-sized resectoscope is not advised. The use of a continuous-flow operative hysteroscope with liquid distention is strongly recommended. Although grade Va adhesions can be treated on an ambulatory basis, they do have a very bad prognosis due to the lack of residual basal endometrium.

In the case of more extensive adhesions, synechiolysis should be performed under general anesthesia and with simultaneous use of other imaging techniques to facilitate the operation and/or prevent complications.

With complete occlusion of the uterine cavity or one of the cornual areas, concomitant laparoscopy must be performed. With transillumination, the laparoscopist can

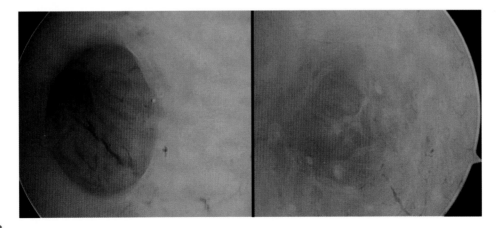

Figure 6.13
(a) A normal tubal ostium. (b) The ostium of the other side at the moment it is closed. Taking the time to check the so-called 'flutter-valve' mechanism of each tubal ostium is important, since it is slow and may mimic an organic stenosis. When the ostium reopens, one also frequently witnesses the passage of small tissue fragments and/or air bubbles that are floating in the saline distention medium towards and through the ostium. If not, a proximal or distal tubal block may be present, and a dye test is then indicated.

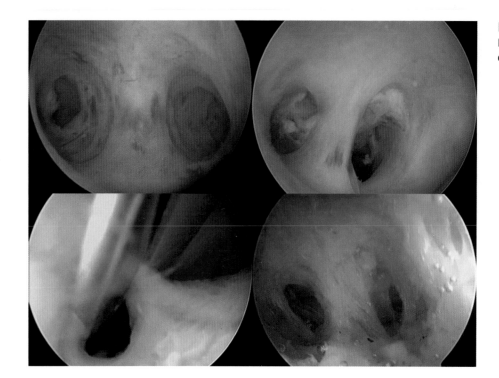

Figure 6.14
Four examples of different degrees of Asherman's syndrome.

guide the hysteroscopist into the right direction and perforation can be avoided as it will be preceded by bright transillumination.

Simultaneous X-ray imaging with intrauterine contrast dye appears to be extremely helpful in cases of extensive adhesions. Small existing openings can be identified and after making a small opening in complete adhesions, the area behind the adhesions can be examined without the need for enlarging the passage.

Abdominal ultrasonography is used by some specialists instead of laparoscopy, in view of the sharp contrast between tissue and distention medium. It can also be applied additionally to identify an adhesion-free, but occluded, part of the uterine cavity which harbors enough functional endometrium. For this purpose, the endometrium can be stimulated with a preoperative treatment of estrogen.

Grade III, IV, and Vb adhesions (see Table 6.5 and Figure 6.13) must be treated under general anesthesia, preferably with laparoscopic or ultrasonographic and/or radiographic control. Synechiolysis in those cases should be performed with conventional operating instruments with a small diameter, high level of brightness, and a wide-angle view. Resectoscopes and lasers are useless in cases of extensive adhesions, as this equipment can easily do more harm than good due to the size of the instruments and/or the lack of 'feeling' (tactile feedback) with the tissue to identify weak spots in the adhesions.

Peroperative antibiotic prophylaxis is recommended.

A continuous and meticulous measurement of the fluid balance of the distention fluid is of vital importance. Intravasation can easily occur during synechiolysis. The fluid 'loss' should never be allowed to exceed 1500 ml to prevent hyponatremia and pulmonary edema. Careful and frequent monitoring of the in/out balance is of the utmost importance in the anesthetized patient. A patient under epidural or rachi anesthesia will get sick with nausea in case of fluid overload.

After synechiolysis some authors leave an IUD (preferably without copper) in the uterine cavity to prevent reocclusion. To enhance regeneration of the endometrium, a 2-month schedule with high-dose estrogen must be prescribed. A control hysteroscopy 2 months after the synechiolysis procedure is highly recommended in severe and difficult cases to treat minor recurrences.

> In cases where there is a suspicion of intrauterine adhesions, blind sounding, dilatation, or insertion of an IUD should never be performed, as there is a high risk in these procedures of creating a false route or even perforation. They often aggravate more than 'treat' the pathology and may reduce the success of subsequent hysteroscopic treatment. The method of choice for both the diagnosis and treatment of intrauterine synechiae is hysteroscopy.

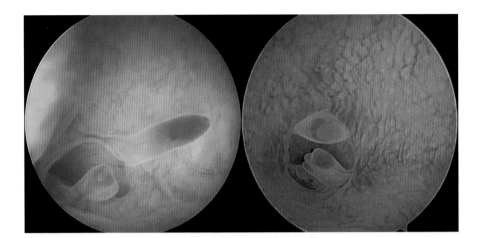

Figure 6.15
Small polyps near the tubal ostium. The clinical significance with regard to the patient's fertility remains to be clarified. Probably, these very small structures are not related to the infertility of the couple.

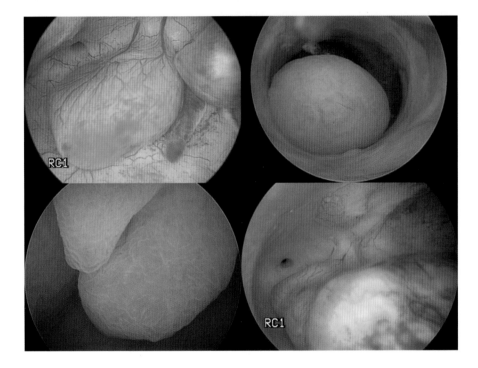

Figure 6.16
Four examples of endometrial polyps, often the cause of spotting or bleeding in between periods but sometimes also including glandulocystic or adenomatous hyperplasia of the polyp's endometrial layer.

Polyps

For therapeutic purposes, one should make a distinction between pedunculated polyps and sessile polyps.

The small pedunculated polyp of soft texture can be removed with mechanical operative hysteroscopy using a small scissors and grasping forceps. The base of the polyp is cut and it is then extracted under visual control. It is also possible to remove these polyps with the resectoscope. In the case of a small polyp, the pedicle is cut, the polyp is grasped with the resection loop and extracted in toto. The tiny polyps one can notice around the tubal ostia (Figure 6.15) are usually left in place, since it is not clear whether or not these polyps are pathologic and, also, their surgical removal may induce a postoperative phimosis or stenosis of the ostium itself.

With larger polyps (Figure 6.16) it would be unwise to cut the stalk of a pedunculated tumor immediately, even if it is very narrow. The polyp, which is then floating inside the cavity, can sometimes not be extracted – due to its size and/or consistency – and it will be even more difficult to cut it into smaller parts once it is no longer fixed to the wall. Therefore, small slices should be cut, progressively removing the polyp.

The sessile polyp is generally better removed with the help of the resectoscope, since it is often not easy to gain access to the broad base of the polyp with scissors. The possibility of movement in only two planes is a limiting factor for mechanical operative hysteroscopy. Before making direct contact with this kind of lesion, it is not always easy to determine if it is a polyp or a myoma. The typical appearance of a polyp during resection is its soft structure and the image of multiple small white spots when cutting through the tissue. They represent the glandular channels or cystic dilated endometrial glands within the polypous structure.

Before surgery, the base of the tumor has to be defined by turning around the lesion using the 30° angle of the optic.

The prominent vessels at the base are first coagulated in order to avoid excessive bleeding and blurring of the vision. Finding the demarcation of and cleavage plane at the base of the polyp can be achieved by gently pushing the resectoscope's loop electrode against its base. This is very helpful, also and especially in the case of hysteroscopic myomectomy. The tumor is then resected progressively by cutting small slices. Although these chips float around or fall down on the posterior uterine wall and can obstruct the surgeon's vision, it is incorrect to take them out after each cut, because moving the resectoscope in and out of the uterine cavity too often increases the risk of air embolism. It is better to remove all the fragments at the end of the procedure or when the view becomes impaired. At the end of the resection, the base of the tumor is coagulated to avoid excessive blood loss. This can be done with the resection loop or with the rollerball.

> For very large sessile polyps it is advisable to remove the superficial part of the entire polyp before entering the myometrium. Indeed, as soon as the removal of the base of the polyp is started at one spot, the risk of fluid overload increases. So it is safer to reserve this part of the resection to the end of the procedure. But nowadays it is preferable to use bipolar loop electrodes together with a physiologic saline solution as a distention medium for the hysteroscopic resection of large polyps and submucous or intramural fibroids, in order to avoid the risk of (hence the need for monitoring) fluid overload and toxicity of anionic solutions such as dextran, glycine, or sorbitol–mannitol (Purisole) altogether.

Endometrial polyps usually lie completely within the uterine cavity and do not extend intramurally. Therefore, they are an ideal structure for the beginner in operative hysteroscopy to train in intrauterine resection as the risk of uterine perforation is usually very low. Resection may occasionally be difficult when a polyp is very mobile and moving away from the cutting loop or when it is located very deeply in the cornual region of the uterine cavity.

Myomas

If an intrauterine myoma is suspected, a diagnostic hysteroscopy should first be performed to evaluate the situation and the type of myoma (see also Table 6.2). With the use of a 30° optic, the exact localization and extension of the myoma is defined by slow rotation. The tubal ostia are also located as helpful landmarks. Sometimes it is not possible to see both ostia, as the myoma may be shadowing one of them. In very large myomas it may even be impossible to gain access to one of the tubal ostia when the myoma is obscuring the view. In the case of profuse uterine bleeding, which is often found in these cases, it can become necessary to use a double-flow hysteroscope to clear the uterine cavity from bloody debris. After diagnostic hysteroscopy, the cervix is dilated to Hegar 8–9.5 (depending on the size of the instrument) for insertion of the resectoscope.

> The use of an 'active type' of working element where, in the 0 position, the loop is out of the working channel, and is brought into the sheath by active pulling with fingers 2–4, seems more physiologic and safer than the use of the 'passive handgrip' where the cutting loop is brought into the sheath by retrograde movement of the operator's thumb.

Type 0 myoma
After again clearly identifying the location of the myoma, the loop is brought behind the myoma, a part of the myoma is 'hooked' on it, and then the loop is pulled through the myoma while activating cutting current.

> A sequential movement, consisting of (1) pulling the loop halfway to the sheath, followed by (2) the retraction of the entire resectoscope, is performed. When doing so, one must follow the outline and curve of the uterine cavity, but this technique allows longer slices to be cut over the whole surface in the case of large myomas (and the same principle can be applied to the endometrial ablation with the cutting loop electrode).

Having cut the first slice, one can usually identify whitish, fibrous tissue as typical for myoma tissue in contrast to the described polyp type of lesion. Systematically, one slice after the other is cut. The chips created are pushed into the cornual region opposite to the myoma. The more chips produced, the more one's vision can become impaired.

The resected chips are best evacuated under direct vision by gently grasping them with the loop electrode and holding them against the optic while removing the whole instrument.

The decrease of distention pressure causes bleeding from the endometrium, the myometrial vessels, and the surface of the remaining part of the myoma. Therefore, after reintroducing the resectoscope, the uterine cavity should first be flushed to allow viewing again; then, resection is continued in a systematic manner until the complete base of the myoma is removed. The resection is followed by careful

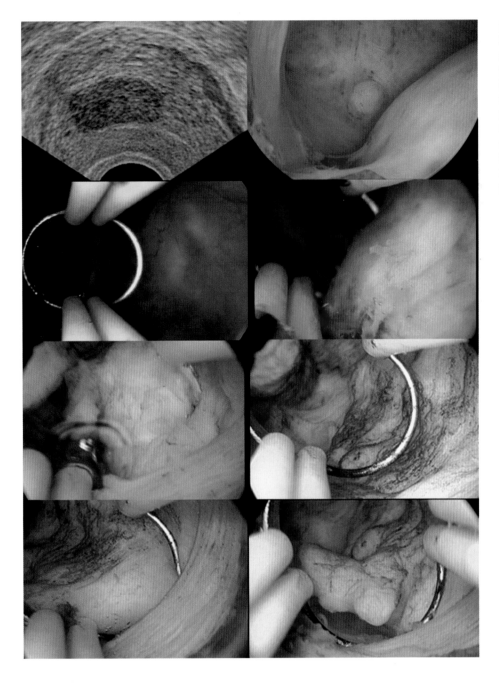

Figure 6.17
Several stages of an operative hysteroscopy for the removal of a type 2 submucous myoma, in this case with the use of a bipolar loop electrode (Karl Storz GmbH, Tuttlingen, Germany) in Hartmann's solution, i.e. without the risk of fluid overload like with macromolecular distention media.

coagulation of the base in order to minimize fluid resorption and to avoid excessive bleeding.

Type I or II myoma

In the case of a type I or type II fibroid it is necessary to carry out a part of the resection inside the uterine wall (Figure 6.17). Usually one can distinguish very well between myoma tissue and normal surrounding myometrium: the myoma has a more dense structure, with whitish color; the myometrium is composed of more connective fibrous tissue with a slightly pinkish appearance.

The deeper the resection is performed into the wall, the greater becomes the risk of uterine perforation. In this situation, one can sometimes enucleate the base of the myoma from its capsule just by blunt dissection. This has the advantage of completing the enucleation without risk of uterine perforation and bowel laceration by the activated cutting loop. This is especially true when vaginal ultrasound indicates a thin safety margin of healthy myometrium and/or when one attempts to resect an intramural fibroid. Only experienced hysteroscopic surgeons can perform these difficult procedures.

In cases with deep intramural resection, it is advisable to interrupt the operative procedure in between to evacuate the cavity. When reintroducing the resectoscope, one can often see that the image has changed completely: the former deep hole in which the base of the myoma is still present now seems to protrude into the uterine cavity and hence can be resected much more easily than before. This may be caused by uterine contractions, and sometimes one can try to further enhance this mechanism by giving drugs, such as oxytocin or ergometrine, that stimulate uterine contractility.

In difficult cases one should consider the performance of simultaneous transabdominal ultrasonography or laparoscopy as safety measures. The hysteroscopic appearance of whitish, bloodless area of tissue or the laparoscopic recognition of white decoloration of the uterine serosa indicate that perforation is likely to occur soon. The residual thickness of the myometrium can be measured exactly by ultrasound.

Although the endoscopic image of bleeding is sometimes very impressive, vaginal bleeding after hysteroscopic myoma resection is only minimal and usually stops within the first 3 postoperative days.

> Hysteroscopic myoma resection usually gives excellent results. Nearly all patients regain eumenorrhea and relief of dysmenorrhea after a minimally invasive procedure that does not cause a great deal of discomfort. Therefore, hysteroscopic resection is the method of choice for the treatment of intrauterine submucous fibroids.

References

1. Campo R, Molinas CR, Rombauts L et al. Prospective multicentre randomized controlled trial to evaluate factors influencing the success rate of office diagnostic hysteroscopy. Hum Reprod 2005; 20: 258–63.
2. Fusi L, Cloke B, Brosens JJ. The uterine junctional zone. Best Pract Res Clin Obstet Gynaecol 2006; Epub.
3. Campo R, Van Belle Y, Rombauts L, Brosens I, Gordts S. Office mini-hysteroscopy. Hum Reprod Update 1999; 5: 73–81.
4. Acién P. Incidence of Müllerian defects in fertile and infertile women. Hum Reprod 1997; 12: 1372–6.
5. The American Fertility Society classifications of adnexal adhesions, distal tubal occlusion, tubal occlusion secondary to tubal ligation, tubal pregnancies, müllerian anomalies and intrauterine adhesions. Fertil Steril 1988; 49: 944–55.
6. Kaufman RH, Adam E, Binder GL, Gerthoffer E. Upper genital tract changes and pregnancy outcome in offspring exposed in utero to diethylstilbestrol. Am J Obstet Gynecol 1980; 137: 299–308.
7. Kaufman RH, Noller K, Adam E et al. Upper genital tract abnormalities and pregnancy outcome in diethylstilbestrol-exposed progeny. Am J Obstet Gynecol, 1984; 148: 973–84.
8. Kaufman RH, Adam E, Hatch EE et al. Continued follow-up of pregnancy outcomes in diethylstilbestrol-exposed offspring. Obstet Gynecol 2000; 96: 483–9.
9. Acién P. Reproductive performance of women with uterine malformations. Hum Reprod 1993; 8: 122–6.

7

Bipolar resectoscope: the future perspective of hysteroscopic surgery

Luca Mencaglia, Emmanuel Lugo, and Cristiana Barbosa

Introduction

The gynecologic resectoscope, born from its urologic equivalent, is commonly used in gynecologic practice to resect or remove intracavitary pathology and also to perform endometrial ablation. The resectoscope consists of a telescope (2.9 and 4 mm, preferably with a 12° angle of view to always keep the loop within the viewing field), an electrical loop to perform passive cuts, and two sheaths for continuous-flow suction and irrigation of liquid distention medium. Besides the cutting loop, other instruments such as microknives or series of coagulation or vaporization electrodes of various shapes can be connected to the resectoscope.

There are essentially two types of resectoscopes which differ in outer diameter: 7.5 mm and 9.2 mm. The 7.5 mm resectoscope should be used in the case of a narrow cervical canal or difficult dilatation, whereas the 9.2 mm resectoscope facilitates the performance of major surgery.[1]

Electrosurgery in hysteroscopy

Biological tissue contains a more or less high concentration of electrolytes, making it sufficiently conductive to be treated by electrosurgery. The thermal effect of high-frequency current is used for separating (cutting) and coagulating tissue (desiccation of tissue). High-frequency (HF) currents must be used on humans, since low-frequency currents can stimulate nerve and muscle cells as a result of electrochemical processes (electrolysis). These effects are small enough to be disregarded with frequencies >100 kHz.[2]

A monopolar or bipolar current system can be adopted.

Monopolar resectoscope

Conventional hysteroscopic surgery uses a monopolar electrocautery system in which the current passes from the active electrode through the patient's body towards the return plate. The distention media used is glycine 1.5% or sorbitol–mannitol (non-electrolyte irrigation fluid). The monopolar resectoscope is connected to a monopolar electrosurgery generator of high frequency, automatically controlled by an acoustic alarm system. In a monopolar system, the electrons flow from an electrosurgery generator to an active electrode (electrode of the loop). From the electrode, the current flow is transmitted to the tissue, then to the plate (neutral electrode), and then it returns to the generator. This system is potentially dangerous since electrons flow through the body, outside the surgeon's visual control, before returning to the generator. The new generators, however, decrease the incidence of electrical damage. In these generators, the cut current flow is automatically regulated by the tissue resistance. The unipolar loop can be used as coagulation, cut and combined (coag-cut) current. The coagulation current/flow is characterized by intermittent current flow periods that cause cellular dehydratation, resulting in tissue emostasis. The non-modulated cut flow is a continuous flow, with high intracellular temperature, causing cellular explosion. Non-modulated flow can be used also for coagulation and should be preferred because the voltage is lower and continuous.[1]

Bipolar resectoscope

In bipolar electrosurgery, the current flow through the tissue is restricted to the area between the two electrode loops that is under visual control of the surgeon. In this case, saline solution can be used as the distention media, because there is no risk of current dispersion. The generator produces a high initial voltage spike that establishes a voltage gradient in a gap between the bipolar electrodes. When the activated bipolar electrode is not in contact with the tissue, the electrolyte solution in the uterus dissipates it. When the loop is sufficiently close to the tissue, the high bipolar voltage spike arc between the electrodes converts the conductive sodium chloride solution into a non-equilibrium vapor layer or plasma effect containing energy-charged sodium particles. Once formed, this plasma effect can be maintained at lower voltages (100–350 RMSV).[3] With tissue contact, there is disintegration of tissue via molecular dissociation. Energetic species of the charged ions from the plasma effect result in disruption of carbon–carbon and carbon–nitrogen bonds. There is also electron impact dissociation of water molecules into exited fragments of H^+ and OH^- ions. The bottom line is rupture of cell membranes, which translates into visible cutting. Clinically, there is a precise tissue effect with minimal collateral damage, as the charged ions have an estimated penetration depth in tissue of only 50–100 μm (0.5–1 mm).[4,5] The depth of coagulation is determined principally by the electrode configuration and by the system design, as well as by the technique used by the operator (time and pressure of contact).[6]

Equipment

The new working element developed by Karl Storz System, the Autocon II 400 (Figure 7.1), is for use in laparoscopy, resectoscopy, and open surgery. It can be equipped with four different HF output sockets: monopolar, bipolar, multifunction, and neutral electrode sockets. The user can assign a socket with the following parameters: cutting mode, coagulation mode, or cutting and coagulation activation type. A mode is characterized by different generator settings such as frequency, peak voltage, and modulation. A total of 10 cutting and 9 coagulation modes are available. However, each specific socket is only available for a part of these modes. The user can also assign the following parameters to a mode: power limitation cutting, cutting effect, power limitation coagulation or coagulation effect.

Using a bipolar system, in the saline time-c-cut mode as the saline coagulation mode, the HF voltage form is unmodulated sinusoidal, the rated frequency is 350 kHz (at RL = 500 ohms) ± 10%, the crest factor is 1.4, the rated load resistance is 50 ohms, the maxim HF peak voltage is 190 Vp, the number of effects available are 8, the maxim power output 300 W ± 20%, and the parameters standard of use are 180 (in effect 4) for cut and 120 (in effect 4) for coagulation. It is important to point out that peak voltages are much lower than monopolar systems.

The bipolar components (Figures 7.2 and 7.3) are compatible with existing resectoscopes (optics, sheath). The sheath, designed by Karl Storz Endoskope, is completely isolated. The direct current returns via the electrode, preventing a current flow via the sheath, and guaranteeing a high level of safety. There are a variety of cutting loops (GP, GPV, GD, GDV) of 24 Fr on the market, but other bipolar loops for resection in gynecology and urology are still being developed.

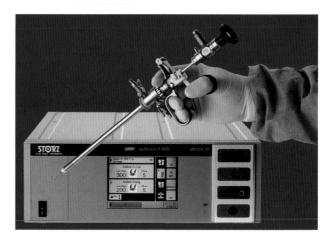

Figure 7.1
Autocon II 400.

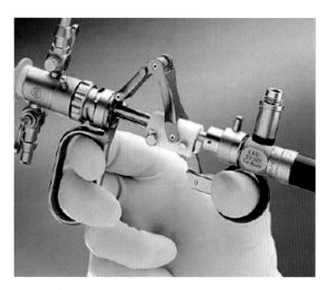

Figure 7.2
The bipolar element of the resectoscope.

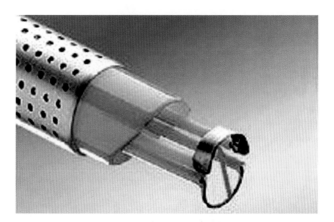

Figure 7.3
The direct current return via the electrode prevents a current flow via the sheath.

Table 7.1 Bipolar resection in 57 patients

Indication	Number of patients	Fibroids >4 cm
Myomas G0	9	1
Myomas G1	15	7
Myomas G2	10	2
Endometrial ablation	12	
Polyps	8	2
Uterine septum	3	2
Total	57	

Clinical data

In 2004, Loffer[7] reported a preliminary experience with the VersaPoint bipolar resectoscope in gynecology. A vaporizing electrode in saline solution distending medium was shown to be effective in removing submucous myomas in 15 patients. Golan et al[8] in 2001 reviewed outcomes of operative hysteroscopy, using bipolar electrical energy (VersaPoint) in saline solution in 116 women with intrauterine pathology. They proposed this new technique as a potential replacement for monopolar resection. Furthermore, many studies have demonstrated the benefits in urology. Recently, Singh et al[9] reported the use of a bipolar system in transurethral prostate resection (TURP) with less postoperative dysuria. In 2004, Wendt-Nordahl et al[10] underlined the advantage of the bipolar system in TURP, with the Vista System, and stressed the theoretical benefit to avoid the risk of the TUR syndrome.

Our preliminary experience in gynecology consists of 57 patients (Table 7.1) treated with a Karl Storz 26 Fr bipolar resectoscope and Autocon II 400 HF unit with parameters standard selected 180 (in effect 4) for cut and 120 (in effect 4) for coagulation. The resection loops are completely insulated from the sheath of the resectoscope and are reusable loops. Saline solution (NaCl 0.9%) was used as distention medium with no complications. Cutting power and coagulation appear better than with monopolar resection. In particular, the first cut in the case of fibroid tissue doesn't give any problem thanks to the plasma effect. Furthermore, the vision during resection is not disturbed by the presence of air bubbles. We included complex cases in our series to evaluate the technical characteristics of the instruments, including an important number of uterine fibroids, that in some cases were >4 cm and G1 and G2 (partially or totally intramural localization). Results in terms of time of surgery, intraoperative bleeding, and complete removal of the pathology were better than with traditional monopolar resection (Figures 7.4–7.7).

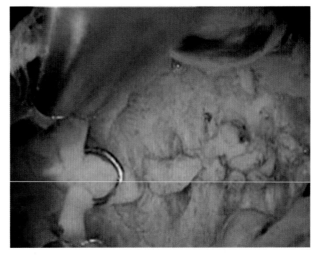

a

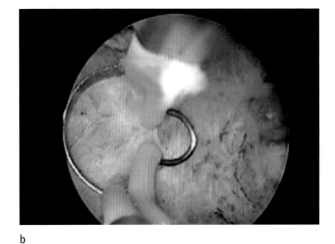

b

Figure 7.5
Metroplasty of uterine septum with bipolar resectoscope.

Figure 7.4
Endometrial polyp resection with bipolar resectoscope.

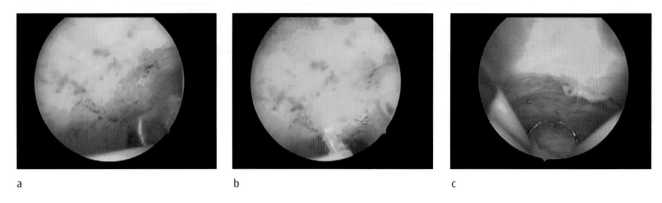

a   b   c

Figure 7.6
Endometrial ablation with bipolar resectoscope.

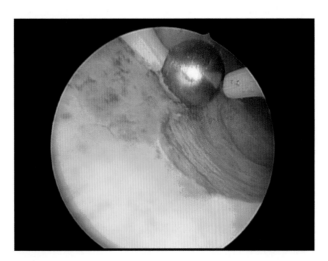

Figure 7.7
Bipolar roller ball.

Conclusion

In our experience, and also in the analysis of the published data, it seems clear that the bipolar resectoscope presents some advantages in comparison with the monopolar resectoscope.

Current flow

The current flow through tissue is restricted to the area between the two electrodes' loops that is under the direct vision of the surgeon. Current can be regulated at all times and set to the lowest possible value: optimal flow of current for minimally invasive treatment. The plasma effect of bipolar current allows better cut and coagulation. In the monopolar technique, the current passes through many tissues outside the surgeon's visual control before it can return to the generator.[5,11] The risk of thermal injuries at distant organs or tissues, by direct contact of instruments, imperfection of insulation, or diffusion of the electric current, is reduced in the bipolar technique.[12,13] It has minor risks of interference with other electronic equipment – electrocardiogram (ECG), pacemakers, etc. – simultaneously connected to the patient.[5,14] Furthermore. there is reduced stimulation of peripheral nerves, including the obturator nerve, because of no flow of current through the body of the patient.

Distention media

According to Kolmer and Norlen[15] and Koshiba et al,[16] the incidence of overflow syndrome in gynecology and TUR syndrome in urology vary considerably in the literature, ranging from 0.18% to 10.9%. Mebust et al[17] reported an incidence of 2% of TUR syndrome in 3885 patients. In 1996, Kudela et al[18] reported the risk of fluid overload syndrome during the hysteroscopy monopolar procedure and underlined the necessity of adhering to safety measures that include selection of a suitable medium (hypotonic electrolyte-free solutions – glycine or sorbitol–mannitol solution), controlling duration of surgery, respecting the correct surgical indications and procedures and, in particular, performing continuous control of the balance of the distention medium. In 2003, Estes and Maye[19] pointed out the danger of hypotonic, electrolyte-free distention media and their potential of being absorbed in volumes large enough to cause hyponatremia and hypervolemia. The main concerns in urologic and gynecologic conventional monopolar resection are fluid absorption with hyponatremia, hypervolemia, and glycine toxicity. This syndrome is very dangerous for the patient, leading to neurotoxic coma and death in the worst cases. Most of the morbidities of the overflow syndrome are related to the use of hypotonic non-electrolyte irrigation fluid. For this reason, close and continuous perioperative monitoring of the balance of the distention medium by a nurse and frequent laboratory investigations are required. The bipolar resection system enables resection using saline solution. The use of saline solution for the distention media of the uterine cavity is the principal advantage of this technology, thus avoiding the use of a hypotonic non-electrolyte solution that can cause fluid overload during the surgical procedure. Saline solution is easily metabolized, is not toxic and can be used with higher quantity, and it is also less expensive than conventional hypotonic non-electrolyte solutions. Singh et al,[9] in a bipolar vs monopolar TURP randomized controlled study, reported a significant difference in serum sodium concentration postoperatively. In bipolar TURP, the change in serum sodium was -1.2 mEq/L (not different from preoperative serum Na concentration), whereas in the monopolar group the mean decrease was 4.6 mEq/L. In three patients serum Na was >125 mEq/L at risk of TUR syndrome. However, the balance of the distention medium using saline solution should also be under control. Starkman and Santucci[20] retrospectively reviewed 43 patients undergoing TURP: 18 consecutive patients treated with monopolar TURP and 25 with bipolar TURP. These investigators found an unexpected case of hyponatremia and pulmonary edema in a bipolar TURP patient. Patel et al[6] also expressed concern for potential problems with hypervolemia and hyponatremia. They suggest warming the saline solution and emptying the bladder from time to time during surgery. In our experience, no overflow syndrome occurs.

Tissue alterations

In traditional monopolar resection, the tissue's electrical resistance creates temperature as high as 400°C, which leads to desiccation with significant collateral and penetrative tissue damage.[6] High-frequency current generated by a bipolar instrument tends to remain superficial; Luciano et al[4,5] reported a 0.5–1 mm depth of penetration compared with the 3–5 mm seen in a monopolar system, allowing a better control of the cut and lower possibility of accidental injury. The technique allows maintenance of the current between the active electrode and the adjacent return electrode. The plasma effect of the loop prevents a sticking effect. In this case, tissue damage is minimized and the tissue temperature range is from 40°C to 70°C. Improved tissue analysis secondary to reduced carbonization of tissue has also been reported with better histologic interpretation. It has also been repeatedly reported that improved visibility aids the identification of surgical landmarks during the procedure.

Less bleeding during resection

Optimized resection current provided by the Autocon II 400 allows a better coagulation during resection, with reduced bleeding. Furthermore, the coagulation capacity, by itself, is much more powerful in the bipolar system than in the monopolar. This avoids time-consuming recoagulation after resection for coagulation and contributes to close the superficial capillary vascularization reducing also intravasation.

Better visibility

Minor air bubbles and less bleeding during resection allow a better vision during surgery, reducing the length of surgery and improving results.

Reduced costs

Compatible components of existing Karl Storz resectoscopes (optics, sheaths) can be used. Only the bipolar element of the resectoscope must be acquired. Resection loops are reusable and have a duration and a cost comparable with the traditional monopolar instruments.

The outcomes of studies in gynecology and urology with the bipolar system demonstrate its versatility and the possibility of rapid replacement of the old monopolar system. The bipolar system is technically superior, cost-effective, and safer compared with the monopolar system. If we take into consideration also the medicolegal aspects, it will be very dangerous to maintain the old system, especially in case of complications. Preliminary findings of decreased morbidity with the bipolar system, using saline solution, force us to consider other factors involved in possible complications, such as duration of the surgery as well as the experience of the surgeon. These variables must be included in our future investigations. However, the decrease of 'theoretical risk' of overflow syndrome that favors the bipolar system does not allow us to avoid close perioperative monitoring of distention medium balance and laboratory investigations.

Larger prospective randomized clinical trails examining cost-effectiveness and long-term outcome need to be performed, although it seems already clear that this technology will replace conventional monopolar electrosurgery in the near future.

References

1. Mencaglia L, Cavalcanti L. Histeroscopia Cirùrgica. Rio de Janeiro: UnionTask Press, 2004: 15–28.

2. Soderstrom RM. Principles of electrosurgery during endoscopy. In: Sammarco MJ, Stovall TG, Steege JF, eds. Gynecologic Endoscopy. Baltimore: Williams & Wilkins, 1996: 179–92.

3. Stadler KR, Woloszko J, Brown IG. Repetitive plasma discharges in saline solutions. Appl Phys Lett 2001; 79: 4503–5.

4. Luciano AA, Whitman G, Maier DB et al. A comparison of thermal injury, healing patterns, and postoperative adhesion formation following CO_2 laser and electromicrosurgery. Fert Steril 1987; 48: 1025–9.

5. Luciano AA. Power sources. Obstet Gynecol Clin N Am 1995; 22: 423–43.

6. Patel A, Adshead J. First clinical experience with new transurethral bipolar prostate electrosurgery resection system: controlled tissue ablation (coblation technology). J Endourol 2004; 18: 959–64.

7. Loffer FD. Preliminary experience with the VersaPoint bipolar resectoscope using a vaporizing electrode in a saline distending medium. J Am Assoc Gynecol Laparosc 2004; 7: 498–502.

8. Golan A, Sagiv R, Berar M, Ginath S, Glezerman M. Bipolar electrical energy in physiologic solution – a revolution in operative hysteroscopy. J Am Assoc Gynecol Laparosc 2001; 8: 252–8.

9. Singh H, Desai M, Shrivastav P, Vani K. Bipolar versus monopolar transurethral resection of prostate: randomized controlled study. J Endourol 2005; 19: 333–8.

10. Wendt-Nordahl G, Hacker A, Reich O et al. The Vista System: a new bipolar resection device for endourological procedures: comparison with conventional resectoscope. Eur Urol 2004; 46: 86–90.

11. Riedel HH, Semm K. There is no place in gynecological endoscope for unipolar of bipolar high frequency current. Endoscopy 1982; 14: 51–4.

12. Levy BS, Soderstrom RM, Dail DH et al. Bowel injuries during laparoscopy. Gross anatomy and histology. J Reprod Med 1985; 30: 168–72.

13. Di Giovanni M, Vasilenko P, Belsky D et al. Laparoscopic tubal sterilization. The potential of thermal bowel injuries. J Reprod Med 1990. 35: 951–4.

14. Odell RC. Electrosurgery: principles and safety issues. Clin Osbtet Gynecol 1995; 38: 610–21.

15. Kolmer T, Norlen H. Transurethral resection of the prostate: a review of 1111 cases. Int Urol Nephrol 1989; 21: 47–55.

16. Koshiba K, Egawa S, Ohori M et al. Does transurethral resection of prostate pose a risk to life? 22-year outcome. J Urol 1995; 153: 1506–9.

17. Mebust WK, Holtgrewe HL, Cockett ATK, et al. Transurethral prostatectomy: immediate and postoperative complications. A cooperative study of 13 participating institutions evaluating 3,885 patients. J Urol 1989; 141: 243–7.

18. Kudela M, Lubusky D, Dzvincuk P. [Risk of fluid overload syndrome during hysteroscopy procedures]. Ceska Gynekol 1996; 61: 291–3 [in Czech].

19. Estes CM, Maye JP. Severe intraoperative hyponatremia in a patient scheduled for elective hysteroscopy: a case report. AANA J 2003; 71: 203–5.

20. Starkman JS, Santucci R. Comparison of bipolar transurethral resection of the prostate with standard transurethral prostatectomy: shorter stay, earlier catheter removal and fewer complications. BJU Int 2005; 95: 69–71.

8

Endometriosis: features at transvaginal laparoscopy

Patrick Puttemans

Introduction

As mentioned in previous chapters of this atlas, the workspace and environment offered by transvaginal hydrolaparoscopy are significantly different from the workspace and working conditions every gynecologist is used to when performing a conventional or standard laparoscopy. First of all, the workspace of transvaginal laparoscopy (TVL) is quite small, meaning that all the organs and tissues, hence all pathologies and lesions, are visualized from a physical distance (i.e. between lens and target) of some millimeters to a couple of centimeters at the most. The images that are obtained in this way can be defined as detailed close-ups that are quite different from the panoramic overview offered by standard laparoscopy. A second difference is the reversed anatomy and topography, not from top to bottom, but exactly the opposite so to speak. The combination of the limited workspace and the reversed approach makes a systematic evaluation of all anatomical regions of the female pelvis very important (Table 8.1). If this systematized way of exploring the pelvis is neglected, then significant lesions of endometriosis may be missed. On the other hand, and

---

Table 8.1 Systematized exploration of the female pelvis via transvaginal laparoscopy

1. Look up the posterior side of the uterus = anatomical landmark at the start of the procedure
2. Go from there to the ovarian ligament and the isthmic part of the Fallopian tube
3. Explore the tubo-ovarian relationship (to rule out the presence of tubo-ovarian adhesions or salpingitis isthmica nodosa)
4. Inspect the whole ovarian surface carefully, using the 30° angle of the optic
5. Explore the ovarian fossa, a common predilection site for endometriosis
6. Turn the optic 180° to explore the uterosacral ligament and the pouch of Douglas
7. Repeat this whole procedure at the other side

---

specifically for endometriosis, the angle at which the ovarian fossa is approached is ideal to explore one of the commonest predilection sites of the disease without any manipulation of the ovary, even in the presence of connecting adhesions between ovary and fossa. This contrasts with standard laparoscopy, where one needs to grasp and rotate the ovary at its ligament in order to visualize the ovarian fossa.

And a third difference is the saline- or Ringer's lactate-filled environment, i.e. a natural, pressure-less and transparent milieu, in contrast to the artificial, gas filled, and pressurized CO_2 pneumoperitoneum at standard laparoscopy.

In view of the features of both peritoneal and ovarian endometriosis described in this chapter, transvaginal hydrolaparoscopy definitely offers a number of advantages over standard laparoscopy, including the recognition of a new and distinct clinical entity in the field of ovarian endometriosis. However, with regard to endometriosis, the technique also presents a number of disadvantages.

Features of endometriosis at transvaginal laparoscopy

The implants

Transvaginal hydrolaparoscopy is a highly accurate technique for the diagnoses of endometriosis and endometriotic adhesions in infertile patients without major pelvic pathology. Inspection under fluid has been reported to improve the visualization of red or 'subtle', non-fibrotic lesions of endometriosis by the three-dimensional optical effect of the fluid environment.[1] These implants have a vesicular or papular form,[2] are sessile or pedunculated yet always turgescent and erect in the aqueous environment (Figures 8.1a–8.1c), and demonstrate a marked increase of the vascularization of the surrounding peritoneum, often with small blood vessels in the stalk and on their surface. Inspection under water ('hydroflotation') facilitates the visualization of these capillary networks within and towards the

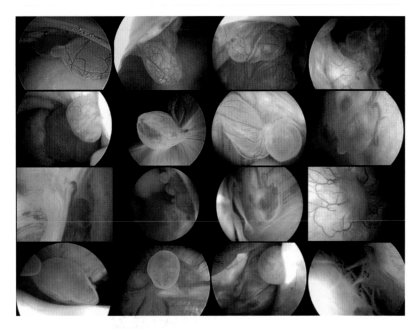

Figure 8.1a
Mosaic of TVL images of active peritoneal endometriosis, once labelled as subtle or atypical. The predilection site for these lesions is the (mostly left) ovarian fossa, the uterosacral ligaments, and the pouch of Douglas. They have a vesicular or papular form, are sessile or pedunculated yet always turgescent and erect in the saline environment, and demonstrate a marked increase of the vascularization of the surrounding peritoneum, often with small blood vessels in the stalk or on their surface.

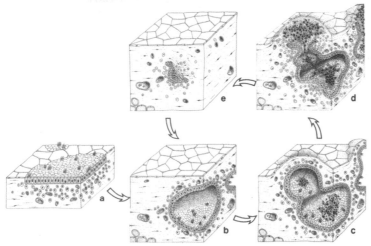

Figure 8.1b
Schematic drawing of what happens in Figure 8.1a: i.e. the cyclic evolution of peritoneal endometriosis: microscopic intramesothelial (a) or submesothelial (b) implants develop into early clinical lesions on the peritoneal surface as distended glands (papules, see c) or glandular polyps (serous or hemorrhagic vesicles, breaking through the mesothelial lining of the serosal surface, see d). These early non-fibrotic lesions may appear and disappear (e) from the peritoneum. The ones that do not disappear may induce adhesions (see Figures 8.5 and 8.6) and/or develop towards a black-blue lesion (see Figures 8.4a and 8.4b). (Reproduced from Brosens et al. Hum Reprod 1994; 9: 770–1[2] with permission from Oxford University Press.)

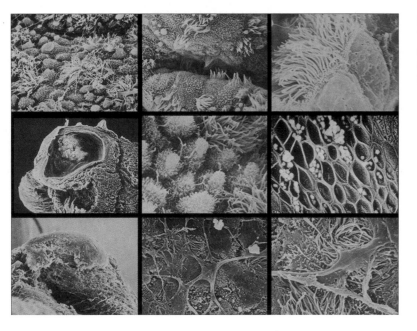

Figure 8.1c
The following SEM (scanning electron microscope) pictures nicely illustrate the ultrastructure of these non-fibrotic peritoneal implants:

  Top row = see Figure 8.1b – drawing (a) and (b)
    glandular epithelium = monolayer of cylindrical ciliated and non-ciliated cells
  Middle row = see Figure 8.1b – drawing (c)
    papule = a distended gland with glandular epithelium at the inside
  Bottom row = see Figure 8.1b – drawing (d)
    vesicle = glandular polyp breaking through the mesothelium

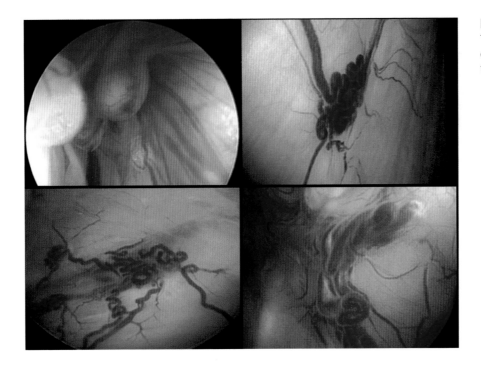

Figure 8.2
Trophic centripetal angiogenesis, often with tortuous blood vessels towards the lesion.

lesions (Figure 8.2), parameters which tend to be masked by the pneumoperitoneum at standard laparoscopy. Figure 8.3 shows the same implants of red, active peritoneal endometriosis, as seen by standard laparoscopy (Figure 8.3a) and as seen by transvaginal hydrolaparoscopy (Figure 8.3b). An inexperienced eye may easily miss the implants on the image in Figure 8.3a, but will never miss them on Figure 8.3b. The classical 'gunshot' or 'powder burn' lesions of endometriosis on the surface of the peritoneum and of the ovary, look exactly the same in a CO_2 pneumoperitoneum as under water (Figures 8.4a and 8.4b).

The adhesions

The systematic inspection of the tubo-ovarian structures under fluid makes it easy to identify filmy, connecting, and

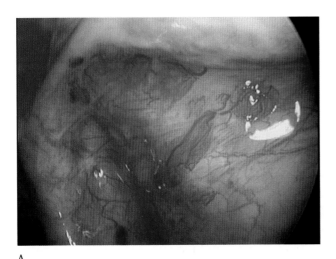

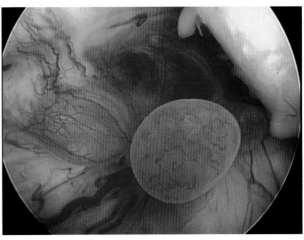

A   B

Figure 8.3
Active peritoneal endometriosis in the left ovarian fossa as seen by standard laparoscopy (a) and as seen by transvaginal hydrolaparoscopy (b). The high-pressure pneumoperitoneum at standard laparoscopy flattens these lesions and if one neglects to inspect the peritoneum at a closer range than merely with a panoramic view, then these active lesions may easily be missed, labeling the infertility of this couple as 'unexplained' if no other factors are present.

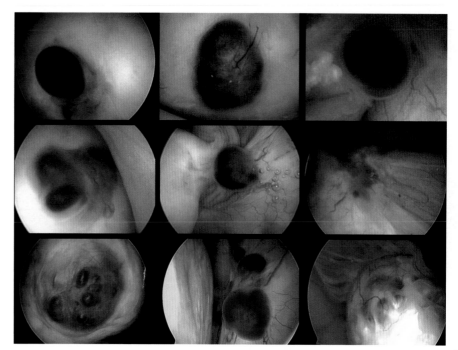

Figure 8.4a
So-called typical 'gunshot' or 'powderburn' lesions of endometriosis, on the surface of the peritoneum and of the ovary. These ovarian lesions can be the 'tip of the iceberg' of a larger and deeper endometrioma, especially when areas of retraction of the ovarian cortex can be seen at the same time. These findings warrant a surgical exploration and, if necessary, extensive bipolar coagulation following the selection of one or more biopsies.

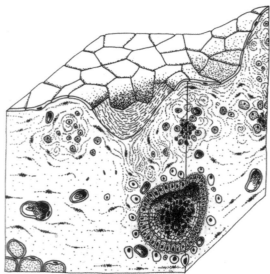

Figure 8.4b
Typical late lesions are the so-called black-blue lesions, which ultimately heal by increasing fibrosis. (Reproduced from Brosens et al. Hum Reprod 1994; 9: 770–1[2] with permission from Oxford University Press.)

non-connecting endometriotic adhesions on the surface of the ovary and peritoneum. The use of saline as the distention medium also provides a remarkable delineation between the ovarian surface and the adhesions.

Unexplained ovarian adhesions were described by Jansen and Russell[3] as subtle endometriosis, but subsequently received little or no attention. Ovarian endometriotic adhesions differ substantially from post-surgical and post-infectious adhesions[4,5] and are characterized by prominent microvascularization (Figure 8.5) and the presence of inflammatory, hemosiderin-laden, endometrial-like cells and fibrin deposits. Subtle endometriotic adhesions are found in 70% of infertile patients with minimal and mild endometriosis at transvaginal hydrolaparoscopy but also in 45% of patients with so-called

'unexplained' infertility. Non-connecting adhesions which may interfere with ovum capture and retrieval by the fimbriae,[6] are seen in 55% of the ovaries in patients with minimal and mild endometriosis and in 36% of the ovaries in patients with unexplained infertility.[7] Comparison of the techniques used to inspect the ovaries showed that standard laparoscopy required the systematic use of an additional instrument to manipulate and expose the inferior or anterior–lateral side of the ovary and the opposing posterior leaf of the parametrium. Traumatic bleeding occurred during that manipulation at standard laparoscopy in 7% of the 43 patients. In contrast, transvaginal hydrolaparoscopy allows for the inspection of the ovaries without any manipulation and detects three times more adhesions than standard laparoscopy. The clinical significance of

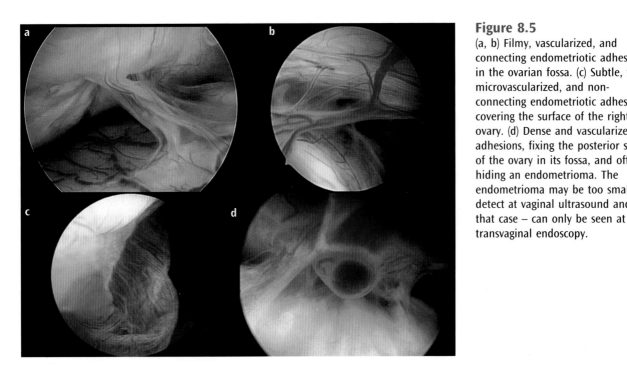

Figure 8.5
(a, b) Filmy, vascularized, and connecting endometriotic adhesions in the ovarian fossa. (c) Subtle, filmy, microvascularized, and non-connecting endometriotic adhesions covering the surface of the right ovary. (d) Dense and vascularized adhesions, fixing the posterior side of the ovary in its fossa, and often hiding an endometrioma. The endometrioma may be too small to detect at vaginal ultrasound and – in that case – can only be seen at transvaginal endoscopy.

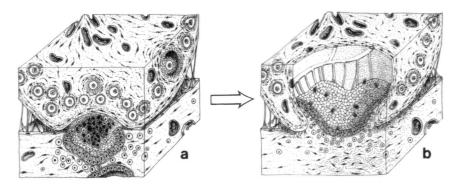

Figure 8.6a
More than 90% of the typical endometriotic (chocolate) cysts form by invagination of the ovarian cortex at the site of the superficial implant, which is encapsulated by adhesions (a). From there, the mucosa-type implant progressively extends over the inverted cortex (b). (Reproduced from Brosens et al. Hum Reprod 1994; 9: 770–1[2] with permission from Oxford University Press.)

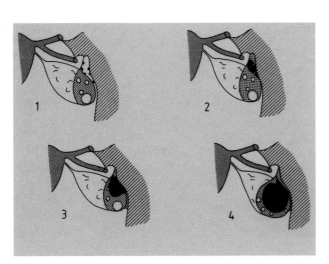

Figure 8.6b
The pathogenesis of the endometrioma starts with peritoneal lesions (1) and adhesion formation (2) in the ovarian fossa and ends with the formation of an entrapped collection of chocolate (3), the growth of which (4) is influenced by three factors: (a) irregular endometrial shedding from the endometriotic lesions inside, (b) retraction, inflammation, erosion, and bleeding from the venules at the hilus of the ovary, and (c) the hindered activity of the ovarian cortex that was invaginated by the whole process, resulting in the development of hemorrhagic functional cysts (not towards the outside of the ovary but towards the inside of the endometrioma) that may contribute signifcantly to the growth of the endometrioma. The endometrioma is in fact a pseudocyst, the inner wall of which does not need to be resected, since it represents invaginated yet in itself normal ovarian cortex containing primordial follicles. Women who have had ovarian cystectomy for endometriomas have systematically fewer oocytes harvested during IVF treatment. Therefore, and especially in the small i.e. young endometrioma, a conservative approach (adhesiolysis, ovariolysis, drainage of chocolate content, biopsies, extensive bipolar coagulation at the inside and at the edges) is indicated and mandatory.

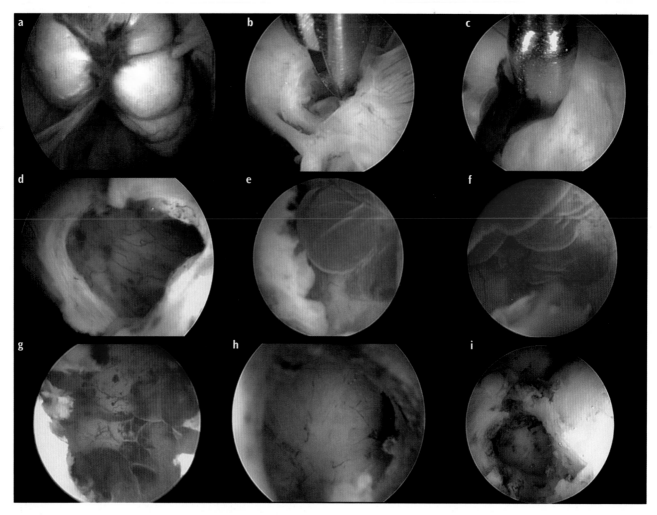

Figure 8.7
The detection, exploration, and treatment of the small endometrioma is feasible via operative TVL. The surgical exploration (b) starts at the zone of retraction of the ovarian cortex (a) or at the site of adhesiolysis between the posterior side of the ovary and the ovarian fossa. The chocolate content is washed out almost automatically by the pressurized infusion of saline at body temperature (c). The optic is then introduced into the endometrioma (d) where one can clearly distinguish the pearl-white ovarian cortex from the superficial mucosa-like endometrium that can easily be pealed off for histology (e, f, and g). The inner surface and the borders of the endometrioma are then coagulated extensively with the bipolar probe (h and i). All visible endometriotic lesions and adhesions on the surface of the ovarian fossa opposite to the endometrioma are also coagulated intensively.

non-connecting adhesions, that are definitely not pathognomonic for endometriosis (other pathologies may induce these subtle inflammatory changes as well), must be clarified by further studies. Sampson[8] and others[9,10] have suggested a primary role of adhesions in the pathogenesis of the ovarian endometrioma (Figures 8.6a and 8.6b).

The endometrioma

The typical features of an endometrioma include:

1. Dense adhesions between the anterior side of the ovary near the hilus and the posterior leaf of the broad ligament or pelvic wall (i.e. what one could call the ceiling of the ovarian fossa).
2. Retraction, scarification, and invagination of the ovarian cortex at the site of the adhesions.
3. The presence of endometriotic lesions and non-connecting adhesions on the surface of the ovary.
4. The entrapment of a variable amount of chocolate.
5. The inner lining of the invaginated cortex inside the endometrioma with mucosa-like implants of red hemorrhagic lesions, the histology of which represents endometrial tissue as a surface epithelium with or without stroma.

These mucosa-type implants (Figures 8.6a, 8.6b and 8.7) are found most frequently at the site of the retraction and adhesion with the parametrium, i.e. endoscopically by the introduction of an optic into the endometrioma.[10] These 'ovarioscopies' and the result of the in-situ biopsies are in agreement with the hypothesis of Hughesdon[9] that 93% of the endometrial cysts originate from invagination of the ovarian cortex (Figures 8.6a and 8.6b). Operative transvaginal hydrolaparoscopy allows for a progressive adhesiolysis/ovariolysis towards the ceiling of the fossa, followed by an incision of the chocolate cyst itself at the site of retraction. The chocolate content will be washed out by the continuous irrigation of saline, and once the vision becomes clear again, the red endometriotic implants can readily be peeled off their pearl-white background for histology and can subsequently be coagulated with the bipolar probe (see Figure 8.7). Currently, the technique is no longer experimental, and endometrial cysts with a diameter ≤4–5 cm can be treated in this way by operative TVL.

The small endometrioma

In an ongoing clinical trial, TVL has proven to be superior to transvaginal ultrasound for the detection of ovarian endometriomas of ≤15 mm in diameter.[11] A total of 564 consecutive women attending the infertility clinic were first investigated with transvaginal ultrasound. Patients without major pelvic pathology were investigated by transvaginal endoscopy that same day. Suspected endometriomas were explored by bipolar dissection and selective biopsies were taken whenever possible. Pelvic endometriosis was detected in 169 patients (29%) at transvaginal hydrolaparoscopy. Cystic ovarian endometriosis was present in 22 of these cases (13%). Transvaginal ultrasound only detected 5 out of 11 endometriomas measuring ≤15 mm in diameter, compared with the detection of 11 endometriomas out of 11 measuring >15 mm in diameter.

There is increasing evidence that the diagnosis of endometriosis, whatever its stage, is important in patients with infertility. The clinical significance of the detection and surgical treatment of small endometriomas in patients with infertility requires further investigation; however, their detection at such an early stage of the infertility exploration and their immediate conservative treatment as a prevention (of further development and growth towards the more severe stages of the disease, with the risk of laparoscopic cystectomy and subsequent premature ovarian failure) definitely deserves our full attention.

Disadvantages of transvaginal laparoscopy with regard to endometriosis

A first and obvious disadvantage of TVL is that not all the areas of the female pelvis are accessible or approachable/reachable by transvaginal hydrolaparoscopy. Endometriotic lesions on the peritoneum of the vesicouterine fold will surely be missed. In a study of 716 women with endometriosis, Koninckx et al[12] found the following anatomic distributions of endometriosis: cul-de-sac and uterosacral ligaments 69%, ovaries 45%, fossa ovarica 33%, and vesicouterine fold 24%. However, isolated peritoneal endometriosis in the vesicouterine fold is very rare and reported to be <4% of cases.[13] So, if one cannot detect any endometriosis by transvaginal hydrolaparoscopy, then the vesicouterine area is probably free of endometriosis as well. Implants within the bladder, however, are within reach of the TVL set of instruments (Figure 8.8).

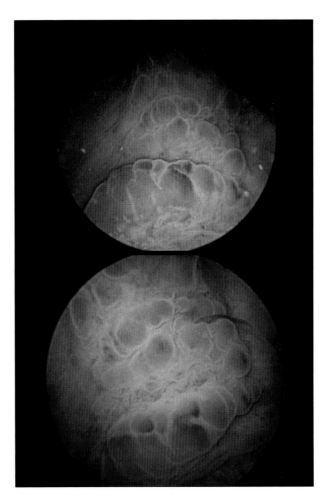

Figure 8.8
An irregularity in the bladder wall near the trigonum at vaginal ultrasound was explored endoscopically ('cystoscopically') using the same optic as the one that is used for TVL. This exploration revealed an endometriotic lesion lifting the bladder mucosa that shows a 'cobblestone' aspect. With the optic locked in the operating sheath (the one we normally use for operative hysteroscopy), a biopsy was taken and the lesion coagulated. Pathologic examination of the biopsy clearly indicated the presence of endometriosis.

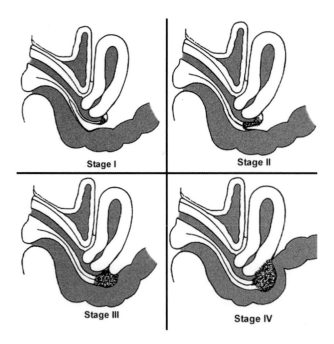

Stage I

Stage II

Stage III

Stage IV

Figure 8.9
When a rectovaginal nodule is felt at clinical examination, this constitutes a major contraindication to perform a transvaginal endoscopy. Since one can never predict if and how the anterior wall of the rectum is involved in this process, the risk of bowel perforation at the insertion of the TVL needle is too high. Thus, deep rectovaginal endometriosis is one chapter of the disease where a TVL cannot be used.

Endometriotic implants on the serosal surface of the bowel may also be missed, since a systematic exploration of bowel loops, e.g. during a laparotomy, is impossible by TVL, as all bowel loops look alike, are floating against each other, and simply cannot be checked over 360° and such a long distance. Endometriotic lesions on rare locations like the diaphragm will also be missed, since TVL can only reach as far as the umbilical region. On the other hand, endometriosis of the appendix has been documented by TVL on a number of occasions, except when adhesions did not allow for a visualization of the appendix itself.

A second disadvantage with regard to the detection and exploration of endometriosis is that deep rectovaginal indurations and nodules constitute a major contraindication to perform a transvaginal hydrolaparoscopy altogether. In such a condition – and that is the reason why a TVL is always preceded not only by a vaginal ultrasound but also by a clinical bimanual examination and even by a rectovaginal examination if in doubt – one can never exclude an abnormally high position of the anterior wall of the rectum in the cul-de-sac, due to dense adhesions with and even involvement of that anterior wall by the process of rectovaginal endometriosis (Figure 8.9). Therefore, the risk of bowel perforation is too high when shooting the needle and inserting the instruments.

Conclusion

Transvaginal endoscopy, performed at an early stage of the infertility exploration, offers a powerful diagnostic tool that provides accurate and reliable information with regard to the detection and staging of endometriosis in the infertile patient without obvious pelvic pathology or with unexplained infertility. Moreover, it also enables us to treat the detected endometriosis efficiently in the majority of cases during that same session.

References

1. Laufer MR. Identification of clear vesicular lesions of atypical endometriosis: a new technique. Fertil Steril 1997; 68: 739–40.
2. Brosens IA, Puttemans P, Deprest J et al. The endometriosis cycle and its derailments. Hum Reprod 1994; 9(5): 770–1.
3. Jansen RPS, Russell P. Nonpigmented endometriosis: clinical, laparoscopic, and pathologic definition. Am J Obstet Gynecol 1986; 155: 1154–9.
4. Jirasek JE, Henzl M, Uher J. Periovarian peritoneal adhesions in women with endometriosis. J Reprod Med 1998; 43: 276–80.
5. Tulandi T, Chen MF, Al-Took S et al. A study of nerve fibers and histopathology of postsurgical, postinfectious, and endometriosis-related adhesions. Obstet Gynecol 1998; 5: 766–8.
6. Gordts S, Campo R, Rombauts L, Brosens I. Endoscopic visualization of the process of fimbrial ovum retrieval in the human. Hum Reprod 1998; 13: 1425–8.
7. Brosens I, Gordts S, Campo R. Transvaginal hydrolaparoscopy but not standard laparoscopy reveals subtle endometriotic adhesions of the ovary. Fertil Steril 2001; 75(5): 1009–12.
8. Sampson JA. Peritoneal endometriosis due to the menstrual dissemination of endometrial tissue into the peritoneal cavity. Am J Obstet Gynecol 1927; 14: 422–69.
9. Hughesdon PE. The structure of the endometrial cysts of the ovary. J Obstet Gynaecol Br Emp 1957; 44: 481–7.
10. Brosens IA, Puttemans PJ, Deprest J. The endoscopic localization of endometrial implants in the ovarian chocolate cyst. Fertil Steril 1994; 61: 1034–8.
11. Gordts S, Puttemans P, Brosens I. Transvaginal hydrolaparoscopy but not transvaginal ultrasound allows detection of small ovarian endometriomas in patients with infertility. Fertil Steril 2004; 82: S338.
12. Koninckx PR, D'Hooghe TD, Oosterlynck D. Response to letter to editor. Fertil Steril 1991; 56: 590.
13. Jenkins S, Olive DL, Haney AF. Endometriosis: pathogenetic implications of the anatomic distribution. Obstet Gynecol 1986; 67: 335–8.

9

Role of transvaginal salpingoscopy

Hiroaki Shibahara, Tatsuya Suzuki, Satoru Takamizawa, and Mitsuaki Suzuki

Introduction

Assessment of the Fallopian tube represents an integral part of the evaluation of the infertile couple. Because the findings obtained at hysterosalpingography (HSG), laparoscopy, or laparotomy are indirect, salpingoscopy has been introduced as an endoscopic examination that can directly evaluate the ampullary tubal mucosa. The standard procedure is transfimbrial salpingoscopy performed at the time of laparoscopy.[1] It is a microendoscopic approach for directly visualizing the tubal mucosa from the ampullary–isthmic junction to the fimbria. Clinical and morphologic studies have shown a high correlation between the appearance of the tubal mucosa and the ultimate outcome in terms of pregnancies.[1] Recently, it was suggested that performing salpingoscopy with laparoscopy could significantly increase accuracy in predicting short-term fertility outcome.[2] However, such salpingoscopy under transabdominal laparoscopy requires hospitalization and general anesthesia.

Transvaginal laparoscopy (TVL) was introduced by Gordts et al to explore the tubo-ovarian structures[3] as well as the ampullary tubal mucosa[4] in infertile patients. We have also been performing TVL and showed its usefulness in investigating infertile women.[5–8] Two advantages of TVL have been shown: it is a less traumatic and more suitable outpatient procedure than transabdominal laparoscopy.

For these reasons, we have been performing TVL for the following five indications: diagnostic TVL[5–8] for (1) tubal obstruction and/or peritubal adhesion are suggested by HSG, (2) serum antibody against *Chlamydia trachomatis* is positive, (3) diagnosis of early-stage endometriosis, and (4) unexplained infertility; operative TVL[9,10] for (5) ovarian drilling using Nd:YAG or holmium laser in infertile women with polycystic ovary syndrome (PCOS).

In some women, endoluminal examination by salpingoscopy can be simultaneously performed under TVL. The transvaginal salpingoscopy under TVL is less invasive to infertile women because it does not require hospitalization or general anesthesia. The procedure was first described by Gordts et al.[4] They reported that the fimbriae were visualized in all patients with no obvious pelvic pathology, and cannulation of the distal tubal segment was achieved without manipulation of the tube in 20% before ovulation and 55% in the early luteal phase. Later, Watrelot et al reported that salpingoscopies were possible in 19% of women with post-PID (pelvic inflammatory disease) lesions without the need to stabilize the tubes. However, salpingoscopies were possible in 41% of those women using a grasp forceps introduced in the operative channel.[11]

We have also been performing salpingoscopy under TVL. Initially, transvaginal salpingoscopy was possible in 13 (18%) of 71 adnexa that were completely visualized.[5] Suzuki et al recently reported the clinical significance of endoluminal assessment by transvaginal salpingoscopy in 130 infertile women.[12] In this chapter, the authors would like to show some findings obtained by transvaginal salpingoscopy using data described in the manuscript.

Transvaginal hydrolaparoscopy and salpingoscopy

Consecutive series of 130 infertile women diagnosed tubo-ovarian structures and tubal passage using TVL (Circon ACMI, Stamford, CT, USA) were retrospectively analyzed between May 1999 and November 2003. The mean age of the subjects was 31.8 years (range: 22–43 years) and the average infertility period was 3.5 years (range: 0.8–15.0 years).

TVL was performed in the lithotomy position as we described previously.[5–10] After disinfection, a Hys-cath (Sumitomo Bakelite Co. Ltd, Tokyo, Japan) was inserted into the uterine cavity for the use of chromotubation. The uterine cervix was lifted with a tenaculum placed on the posterior lip and the central part of the posterior fornix was infiltrated with 2 ml of 1% lidocaine. A Veress needle was introduced 1.5 cm below the cervix and inserted into the pelvic cavity. Approximately 100 ml of saline was instilled in the pouch of Douglas. A 3 mm blunt trocar was inserted

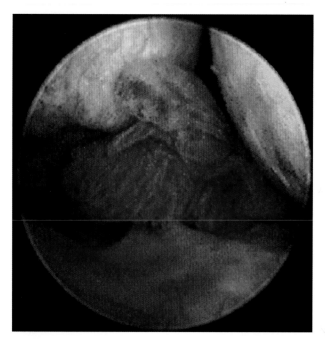

Figure 9.1
The posterior of the uterus and the bilateral tubo-ovarian structures were carefully observed by TVL. The ovary and fimbriae are clearly visible.

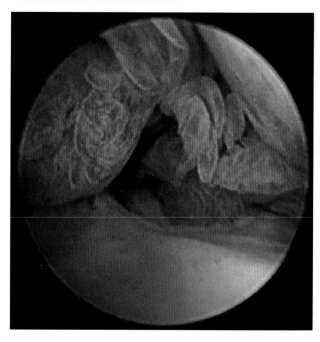

Figure 9.2
A view of the normal-looking fimbriae by TVL.

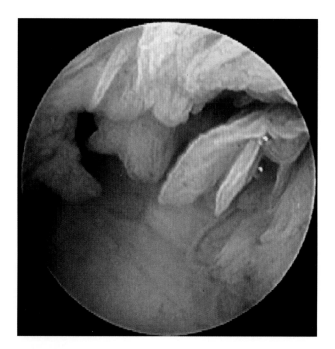

Figure 9.3
Tubal passage was confirmed using indigo carmine. A Hyscath was inserted into the uterine cavity for the use of chromotubation.

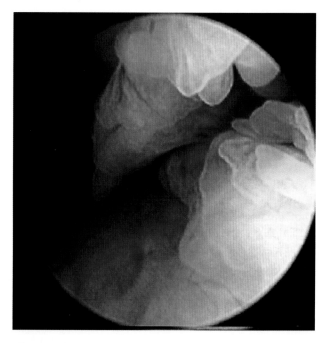

Figure 9.4
Chromotubation was useful to the operator to identify the fimbria.

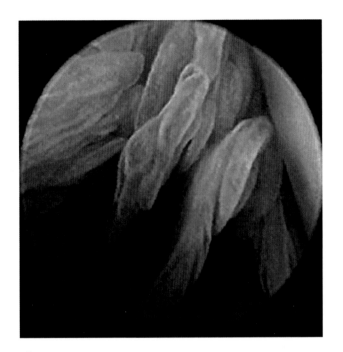

Figure 9.5
The endoscope was inserted from the fimbria by the guidance of chromotubation.

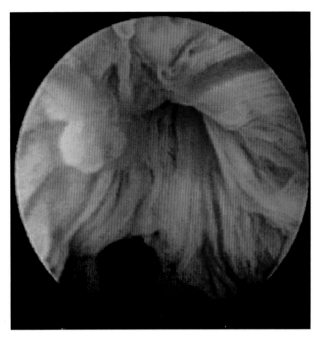

Figure 9.6
The endoscopic finding of the normal-looking fimbria.

by a stab incision in the posterior fornix and then a 2.7 mm diameter semirigid endoscope was used at an optical angle of 30° and a flow channel attached to a 3-CCD digital video camera. The saline irrigation was continued throughout the procedure to keep the bowel and tubo-ovarian structures afloat. The posterior of the uterus and the bilateral tubo-ovarian structures were carefully observed (Figures 9.1 and 9.2), and tubal passage was confirmed using indigo carmine (Figures 9.3 and 9.4).

Salpingoscopic findings

TVL was carried out in 130 infertile women in the study period. Access to the pouch of Douglas was achieved in 123 (94.6%) of 130 patients. Twenty-six tubes could not be visualized because of extensive adhesion. Two patients with a history of unilateral salpingectomy and a patient with unicorn uterus were excluded. Therefore, 217 adnexa were clinically evaluated.

In 89 (41.0%) of 217 tubes, a salpingoscopy could be performed. The endoscope was inserted from the fimbria (Figures 9.5 and 9.6) by the guidance of chromotubation (Figure 9.7) and the distal part of the tubal mucosa could be observed (Figures 9.8–9.14). This result is similar to the first report of transvaginal salpingoscopy by Gordts et al,[4] who reported that the distal tubal segment was cannulated

successfully without additional instrumentation in 47%. To increase the success of salpingoscopy rates, it may be necessary to stabilize the tubes using grasp forceps to introduce an operative channel demonstrated by Watrelot et al.[11]

Each tubal finding under TVL was assigned to one of three classes, comprising regular, convoluted, and hydrosalpinx, as shown in Table 9.1.[13] Tubal obstruction was diagnosed in 36 (16.6%) of the 217 tubes, whereas convoluted tubes or hydrosalpinges were diagnosed in 102 (47.0%) of the 217 tubes. A salpingoscopy could be performed in 87 (48.1%) of 181 patent tubes, significantly higher than that of 2 (5.6%) in 36 obstructed tubes (p <0.0001). A salpingoscopy was easily performed in patent tubes because chromotubation allowed the operator to identify the fimbrial ostium easily. It was also successfully

Table 9.1 Classification of laparoscopic findings

Regular	normal morphology
Convoluted	any altered morphology except for hydrosalpinx
Hydrosalpinx	dilated tube with distal occlusion

Reproduced from Marchino et al,[13] with permission.

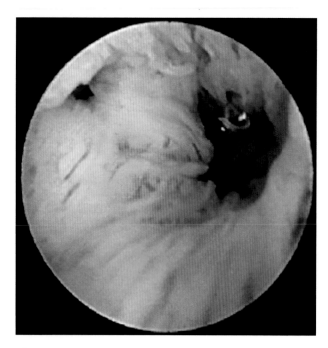

Figure 9.7
The endoscope was inserted into the ampulla by the guidance of chromotubation.

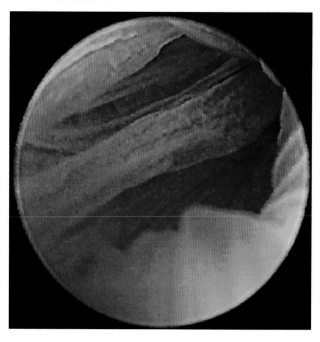

Figure 9.8
The distal part of the tubal mucosa was observed.

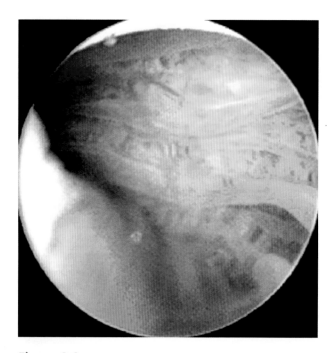

Figure 9.9
The normal-looking tubal mucosa under transvaginal salpingoscopy.

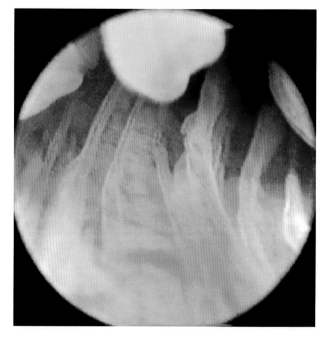

Figure 9.10
The ampullary mucosa was clearly visible.

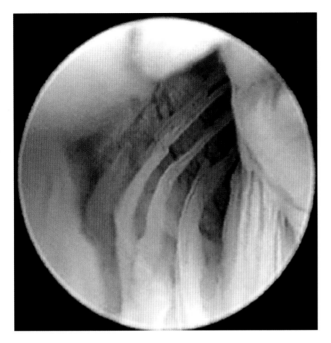

Figure 9.11
The salpingoscope was deeply inserted into the ampulla.

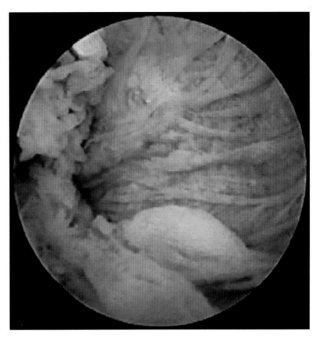

Figure 9.12
Chromotubation finding in the normal tubal mucosa.

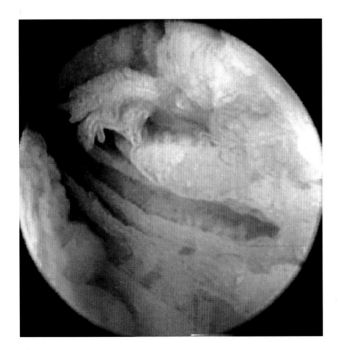

Figure 9.13
The normal-looking tubal mucosa.

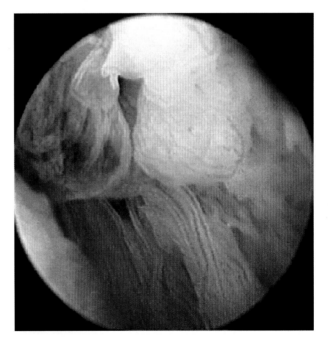

Figure 9.14
The normal-looking tubal mucosa.

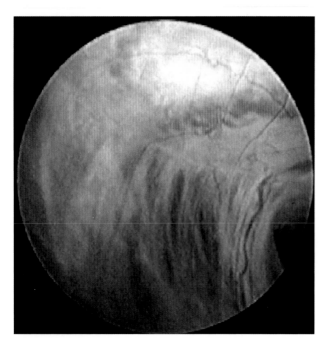

Figure 9.15
Unsuccessful salpingoscopy in a case of extensive peritubal adhesion by previous *C. trachomatis* infection.

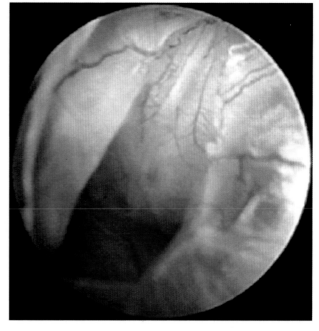

Figure 9.16
Extensive peritubal adhesion by previous *C. trachomatis* infection.

performed in 55 (47.8%) of 115 regular tubes, which was significantly higher than that of 34 (33.3%) in 102 convoluted tubes or hydrosalpinges ($p = 0.03$). Deformed fimbriae or fimbrial adhesions prevented the cannulation of the distal tubal segment.

However, a history of *C. trachomatis* infection did not always influence the success of a salpingoscopy, because extensive peritubal adhesion by previous *C. trachomatis* infection may disturb visualizing the tubes themselves (Figures 9.15–9.17). Therefore, we speculate that the successful salpingoscopy rate was similar between women with and without previous *C. trachomatis* infection. Typical tubal damage by *C. trachomatis* infection includes verruca and atypical vessel formation, peritubal adhesion, and endosalpingial edema (Figures 9.18–9.20).

The correlation between laparoscopic and salpingoscopic findings remains controversial. In the present study, the 89 tubes that were observed by a salpingoscopy, were divided into three categories according to the laparoscopic findings as described above: regular 53 (59.6%); convoluted 34 (38.2%), and hydrosalpinx 2 (2.2%). They were also divided into five categories according to the salpingoscopic findings according to Puttemans et al,[14] as shown in Table 9.2: grade I 66 (74.2%), grade II 19 (21.3%), grade III 3 (3.4%), grade IV 1 (1.1%), and grade V 0 (0%). Statistical analysis demonstrated a significant correlation between salpingoscopic and laparoscopic findings ($r = 0.50$; p <0.0001). These data were supported by the previous

Table 9.2 Classification of salpingoscopic findings

Grade I	normal folds
Grade II	distended fold pattern
Grade III	focal lesions (adhesions, polyps, stenosis)
Grade IV	extensive lesions with or without destruction of mucosa
Grade V	complete loss of mucosal fold pattern

Reproduced from Puttemans et al,[14] with permission.

reports demonstrating a positive correlation between salpingoscopic and laparoscopic findings.[15,16] On the contrary, several groups arrived at the opposite conclusions.[14,17,18] We consider that TVL and salpingoscopy should be simultaneously performed if possible in order to refer to the determination of the next treatment strategies.

Role of transvaginal salpingoscopy

We previously reported the usefulness and prognostic value of TVL in infertile women, and concluded that TVL

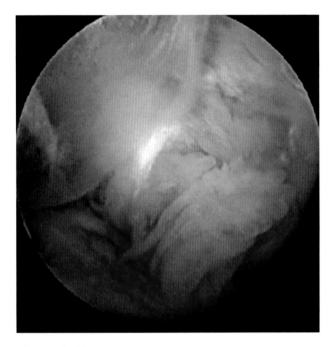

Figure 9.17
Disturbance of visualization of the tubes due to previous *C. trachomatis* infection.

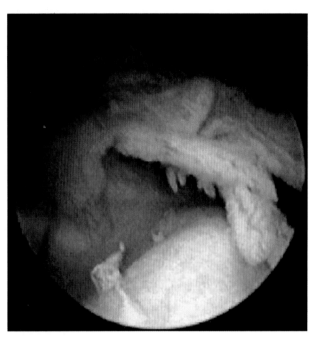

Figure 9.18
Typical tubal damage by *C. trachomatis* infection. Ischemic appearance of fimbria.

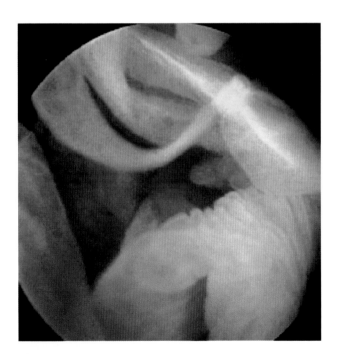

Figure 9.19
Peritubal adhesion by *C. trachomatis* infection with normal chromotubation.

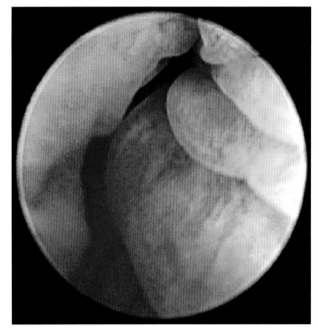

Figure 9.20
Endosalpingial edema caused by *C. trachomatis* infection.

is useful in selecting a future treatment strategy.[5,6] Women with severe tubal disease were recommended in vitro fertilization–embryo transfer (IVF-ET).

In this study, 16 patients who experienced a salpingoscopy bilaterally were carefully monitored for at least 6 months with appropriate infertility treatment, excluding IVF-ET. Pregnancies were established in 10 (62.5%) of 16 patients, with four pregnancies by timed intercourse and six by artificial insemination with the husband's sperm (AIH). Tubal pregnancies were not included. The number of pregnancies did not differ between patients with regular and those with convoluted tubes. For example, four pregnant women (80%) with salpingoscopic grade I tubes had a convoluted tubal appearance at laparoscopy. This indicates that the salpingoscopy may be a better predictor of future fertility outcome than TVL alone. Previous reports also suggested that the simultaneous performance of salpingoscopy and laparoscopy could predict the reproductive outcome better than laparoscopy alone.[2,15–19]

In conclusion, these findings suggest that endoluminal assessment by transvaginal salpingoscopy can be simultaneously performed in some infertile women, especially with patent tubes or with regular tubes undergoing TVL. Further studies are being carried out to clarify the usefulness of intratubal exploration as a tubal infertility assessment.

References

1. Brosens I, Boeckx W, Delattin P et al. Salpingoscopy: a new pre-operative diagnostic tool in tubal infertility. Br J Obstet Gynaecol 1987; 94: 768–73.
2. Marchino GL, Gigante V, Gennarelli G et al. Salpingoscopic and laparoscopic investigations in relation to fertility outcome. J Am Assoc Gynecol Laparosc 2001; 8; 218–21.
3. Gordts S, Campo R, Rombauts L, Brosens I. Transvaginal hydrolaparoscopy as an outpatient procedure for infertility investigation. Hum Reprod 1998; 13: 99–103.
4. Gordts S, Campo R, Rombauts L, Brosens I. Transvaginal salpingoscopy: an office procedure for infertility investigation. Fertil Steril 1998; 70: 523–6.
5. Shibahara H, Fujiwara H, Hirano Y et al. Usefulness of transvaginal hydrolaparoscopy in investigating infertile women with *Chlamydia trachomatis* infection. Hum Reprod 2001; 16: 1690–3.
6. Fujiwara H, Shibahara H, Hirano Y et al. Usefulness and prognostic value of transvaginal hydrolaparoscopy in infertile women. Fertil Steril 2003; 79: 186–9.
7. Shibahara H, Hirano Y, Ayustawati et al. Chemokine bioactivity of RANTES is elevated in the sera of infertile women with past *Chlamydia trachomatis* infection. Am J Reprod Immunol 2003; 49: 169–73.
8. Shibahara H, Takamizawa S, Hirano Y et al. Relationships between *Chlamydia trachomatis* antibody titers and tubal pathology assessed using transvaginal hydrolaparoscopy in infertile women. Am J Reprod Immunol 2003; 50: 7–12.
9. Hirano Y, Shibahara H, Takamizawa S et al. Application of transvaginal hydrolaparoscopy for ovarian drilling using Nd:YAG laser in infertile women with polycystic ovary syndrome. Reprod Med Biol 2003; 2: 37–40.
10. Shibahara H, Hirano Y, Kikuchi K et al. Postoperative endocrine alterations and clinical outcome of infertile women with polycystic ovary syndrome after transvaginal hydrolaparoscopic ovarian drilling. Fertil Steril 2006; 85: 244–6.
11. Watrelot A, Dreyfus JM, Andine JP. Evaluation of the performance of fertiloscopy in 160 consecutive infertile patients with no obvious pathology. Hum Reprod 1999; 14: 707–11.
12. Suzuki T, Shibahara H, Hirano Y et al. Feasibility and clinical significance of endoluminal assessment by transvaginal salpingoscopy under transvaginal hydrolaparoscopy in infertile women. J Minim Invasive Gynecol 2005; 12: 420–5.
13. Marchino GL, Gigante V, Gennarelli G et al. Salpingoscopic and laparoscopic investigations in relation to fertility outcome. J Am Assoc Gynecol Laparosc 2001; 8: 218–21.
14. Puttemans P, Brosens I, Delattin P et al. Salpingoscopy versus hysterosalpingography in hydrosalpinges. Hum Reprod 1987; 2: 535–40.
15. Marana R, Rizzi M, Muzii L et al. Correlation between the American Fertility Society classifications of adnexal adhesions and distal tubal occlusion, salpingoscopy, and reproductive outcome in tubal surgery. Fertil Steril 1995; 64: 924–9.
16. Surrey ES, Surrey MW. Correlation between salpingoscopic and laparoscopic staging in the assessment of the distal fallopian tube. Fertil Steril 1996; 65: 267–71.
17. De Bruyne F, Hucke J, Willers R. The prognostic value of salpingoscopy. Hum Reprod 1997; 12: 266–71.
18. Marana R, Catalano GF, Muzii L et al. The prognostic role of salpingoscopy in laparoscopic tubal surgery. Hum Reprod 1999; 14: 2991–5.
19. Heylen SM, Brosens IA, Puttemans PJ. Clinical value and cumulative pregnancy rates following rigid salpingoscopy during laparoscopy for infertility. Hum Reprod 1995; 10: 2913–16.

10

Operative transvaginal laparoscopy

Stephan Gordts

Introduction

The technique of diagnostic transvaginal laparoscopy (TVL) as an outpatient procedure was described by us for the first time in 1998.[1,2] It was meant to offer the subfertile patient without obvious pelvic pathology the possibility of a minimally invasive endoscopic exploration of the pelvis.

As a distention medium, pre-warmed Ringer's lactate is used; it contributes to an accurate and correct visualization and to floating of the organs. Consequently, tubo-ovarian structures can be inspected in their natural position without supplementary manipulation.

After gaining more experience with the technique, it became obvious that the easy access to the ovarian surfaces, the fossa ovarica, and the Fallopian tubes opened the potential for some operative procedures. With the endoscopic instruments in the same axis, the transvaginal approach creates excellent possibilities for a minimally invasive dissection of the ovary under direct vision.

Technique and instruments

As for the diagnostic procedure, the patient lies in a dorsal decubitus position and access to the pelvis is gained through the same needle puncture technique. After verification of the correct localization of the diagnostic instruments, a specially developed obturator allows easy exchange between the diagnostic and the operative instruments (Figure 10.1). A 2.9 mm endoscope with a 30° optical angle is inserted in

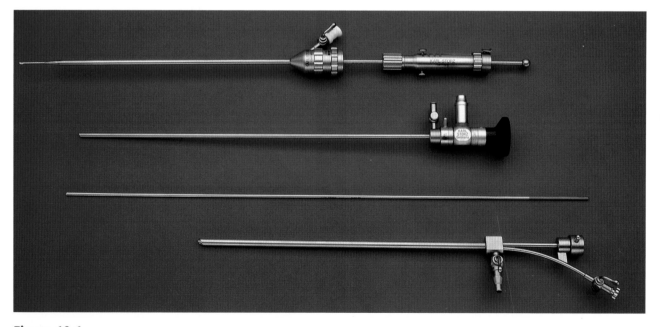

Figure 10.1
Set for transvaginal endoscopy, showing:
* the assembled needle
* the 2.9 mm endoscope with the diagnostic trocar of 3.7 mm
* the obturator allowing a switch from the diagnostic sheet to the operative sheet
* the operative trocar with one channel.

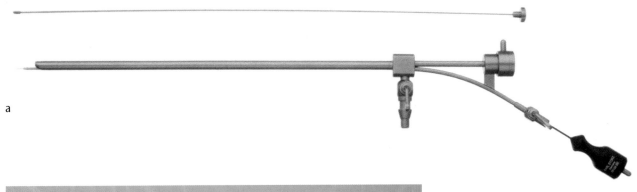

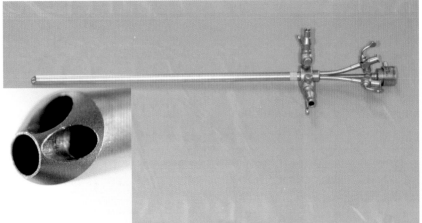

a

b

Figure 10.2
The operative trocars: (a) one channel with the bipolar needle; (b) two channels allowing the introduction of 5 Fr instruments.

the operative trocar sheet with one or two operative channels (Figure 10.2), with outer diameters of 5 and 7 mm, respectively. The operative channels allow the insertion of 5 Fr instruments such as scissors, biopsy, and grasping forceps and bipolar coagulation probes. The two-channel operative trocar is mostly used in the case of ovarian endometrioma, as it allows the insertion of the bipolar probe through one channel and scissors or forceps through the other one.

Before starting the procedure, about 100 ml of warm Ringer's lactate is instilled in the pouch of Douglas to give the necessary distention.

As we are working in an aqueous distention medium, preventive and meticulous hemostasis with bipolar coagulation is mandatory to avoid insufficient or disturbed view. During the entire procedure, a continuous flow of prewarmed Ringer's lactate is used.

Although tubo-ovarian structures are easy accessible, the lack of panoramic view will restrict the technique to minor operative procedures. The technique is indicated in cases of superficial peritoneal and ovarian endometriosis, small endometriomas, tubo-ovarian adhesiolysis, and drilling of ovarian capsule in cases with clomiphene-resistant polycystic ovaries. Acute situations such as intra-abdominal bleeding or infection are an absolute contraindication.

Superficial endometriosis and ovarian endometrioma

About 50–60% of the pathologic findings at TVL are due to the presence of superficial endometriosis.[3] These lesions are mostly associated with free-floating ovarian or peritoneal adhesions or fixed adhesions with the fossa ovarica. The findings at TVL correspond very well with the regurgitation and implantation theory of Sampson[4] followed by adhesions and invagination of the ovarian cortex, as demonstrated by Hughesdon and Brosens[5,6] (Figure 10.3). Therefore the endometriosis in an ovarian endometrioma is superficial, as it is lining the invaginated cortex. The access to the ovary is achieved without manipulation, since there is a direct exposure of the fossa ovarica. At this site, endometrioma are frequently adherent to the lateral pelvic wall, the uterosacral ligament. or the posterior leaf of the broad ligament.

The technique for reconstructive ovarian surgery (Figure 10.4) at TVL is based upon the same principles as at standard laparoscopy (SL): the first step consists of an adhesiolysis with full mobilization of the ovary and identification of the site of inversion; at the second step, the cyst is opened at the site of inversion. Access into the endometriotic cyst at

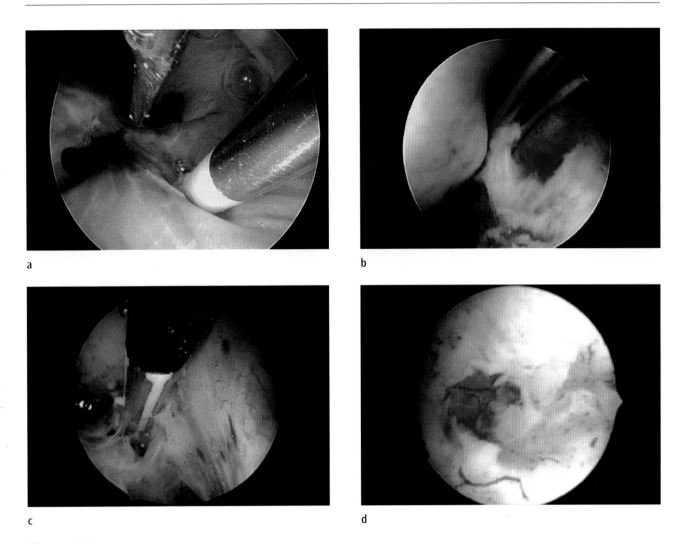

Figure 10.3
(a) Dissection and opening of a superficial peritoneal lesion using the bipolar probe and scissors. (b) After removal of the superficial peritoneal adhesions, endometrial-like tissue can be visualized at the base of the lesion. (c) A 5 Fr bipolar probe used for coagulation and dissection. (d) Partial coagulated small endometrioma: note the invagination of the cortex, with, at the base, still the presence of some neovascularization, and the non-collapsing of the walls.

this side is essential to minimize ovarian trauma and to maintain patency of the pseudocyst. This technique differs from fenestration, as the opening of the pseudocyst is performed by adhesiolysis and resection of the fibrotic ring at the site of inversion. After aspiration and rinsing, the site of inversion is widely opened. At the third step, a superficial and abrasive coagulation is performed of the vascularized endometriotic lesions lining the wall.[7] Because of the watery distention medium and in the absence of a high intra-abdominal pressure, the neoangiogenesis remained visible, facilitating the identification of endometrial implants. We found no difference in recurrence rate of endometriomas between microsurgical resection of the wall and the present simplified technique of eversion or marsupialization and coagulation.[8] In the case of an endometrioma >5 cm, the

treatment was performed in two steps. This is also our normal strategy in the case of a classical operative laparoscopy.[9] During the first procedure, adhesiolysis with resection of the fibrotic area at the site of inversion is performed with coagulation of the visible vascularized endometriotic implants. During the second step, adhesiolysis is performed whenever necessary and the fulguration of the reduced pseudocyst is completed. Our preliminary results showed no recurrence of an endometrioma in operated patients with a follow-up of 12–36 months. After opening of the endometrioma, there is no collapse of the wall as this is formed by the rigid ovarian cortex; this is in contrast with true intraovarian cysts (Figure 10.4e).

In our series of operative TVL procedures, no conversion to laparoscopy was necessary. Compared with the

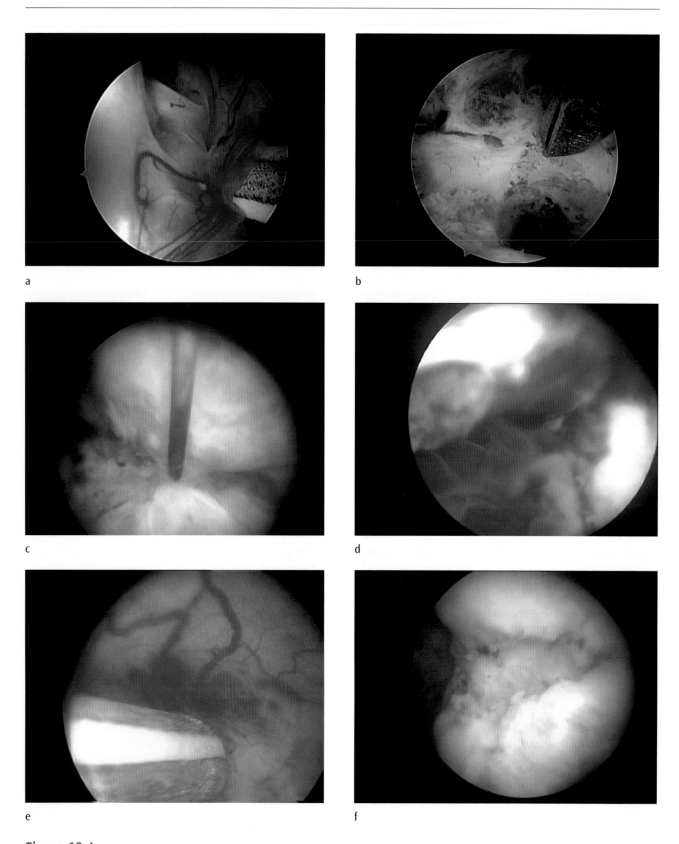

Figure 10.4

Technique for reconstructive ovarian surgery. Dissection of fossa ovarica using the (a) bipolar probe and (b) scissors. (c) A bipolar needle is used for incision of the endometrioma at the place of invagination. (d) After opening, endometrial-like tissue is clearly visible at the base of the pseudocyst. (e) A bipolar probe is used for coagulation. Invagination is clearly visible after coagulation with the bipolar probe. (f) After coagulation, no carbonization occurs.

morbidity after an SL, the morbidity after the transvaginal procedures was very low and most of the patients had no sensation of pain afterwards and at most complained of a light tenderness in the lower abdomen. All patients returned home the same day and resumed their full activity 1 or 2 days later. The 1-day hospitalization and the low morbidity of the procedure makes a second-step procedure also more acceptable for the patient.

The underwater inspection of small ovarian endometriotic lesions confirms the invagination theory of Hughesdon and Brosens.[5,6] What initially appear as small brown superficial ovarian lesions reveal at closer inspection to be invaginated areas of the ovarian cortex covered by small adhesions. After opening and at the base of these invaginated areas, typical endometrial-like implants with their neovascularization can be identified (Figures 10.3 and 10.4).

The disadvantage that was noted during the pioneering years does not apply to the same extent today: with time, experience, and a constant effort on behalf of the manufacturing company (Karl Storz, Tüttlingen, Germany) to provide ever-better prototypes of the instruments, operative TVL now allows us to treat stage I, II, and even specific cases of stage III endometriosis of the adnexa. However, some limitations are still present:

1. Despite the availability of a very efficient bipolar coagulation probe, a problem with hemostasis, i.e. uncontrolled bleeding of blood vessels, might occur and blur the vision in such a way that it becomes impossible and dangerous to continue the procedure. The chocolate content of an endometrioma, however, is not a cause of a blurred vision, since it is washed out quite efficiently by the pressurized infusion of Ringer's lactate.
2. The inability to expose cleavage planes between different types of tissue in the same way as with the help of an assistant or resident during operative laparoscopy via three or four suprapubic ports; here, the surgeon is alone and has to rely mostly on the visual information coming from the operating field. There is also, but to a much lesser degree, some form of tactile feedback when touching tissues. Prototypes of operating sheaths with two (instead of one) operating channels proved to be very promising since one channel can then be used to hold or fix tissue planes, while the other channel serves to operate (take a biopsy, incise, excise, coagulate, etc.)
3. The progress during operative TVL with the current instruments is still more time consuming than during a conventional operative laparoscopy; one can only proceed at the pace of millimeters rather than of centimeters.

This means that, at this moment, it is probably wiser and less time consuming, even with a vast surgical experience, to treat ovarian endometriomas of >40–50 mm in diameter by conventional operative laparoscopy. Nevertheless, operative transvaginal hydrolaparoscopy is definitely the ideal tool to detect and treat the small ovarian endometrioma of ≤15 mm, meaning that in most of these instances the detection of such a small endometrioma will always be followed by its treatment during that same procedure.

Ovarian capsule drilling

The TVL is also very suitable for performing drilling of the ovarian capsule in patients with polycystic ovary syndrome (PCOS) resistant to medical therapy. One of the major concerns of laparoscopic drilling of the ovaries was the risk of postoperative adhesion formation. The CO_2 pneumoperitoneum has been shown to induce acidosis and enhance adhesion formation by its deleterious effect on the oxygenation of the peritoneal mesothelial layers.[10] Although further examinations are necessary to prove the diminished risk of adhesion formation if procedures are performed under water using a pre-warmed solution of Ringer's lactate as a distention medium, data from experimental work in mice has shown that less adhesions were induced if the same surgical procedure was performed under water compared with the use of a pneumoperitoneum with CO_2.[11,12]

After identification of the ovarian surface, drilling of the ovarian capsule is performed using a bipolar needle with a diameter of 1 mm and a length of 0.8 cm (Figure 10.5a). The needle is placed perpendicular to the ovarian surface and is gently pushed against the ovarian surface (Figure 10.5b and c). The capsule is perforated using a bipolar cutting current, allowing an easy insertion of the needle. A coagulating current is used for 5 seconds, followed by the removal of the needle. Although there are no data available with regard to the numbers of holes to be performed, our policy is to make about 10–15 small holes on each ovarian surface, preferentially on the anterolateral site (Figure 10.5d). When the current is switched on, the continuous flow of Ringer's lactate is stopped, allowing a more accurate performance of the bipolar current and a maximal effect of energy delivery. The total procedure doesn't last longer than 30 minutes. The small needle diameter minimizes the defect on the ovarian capsule and, in the absence of carbonization in a watery environment, risks for postoperative adhesion formation will be reduced.

Our results are in line with the results of others[13,14] and are comparable with those obtained after drilling through SL.[15] Restoration of monofollicular cycles, avoidance of multiple pregnancies, and the higher risks for complications are all factors in favor of a surgical treatment of PCOS. At the same time, a complete exploration of the female pelvis can be carried out. In the absence of the postoperative onset of ovulatory cycles, ovulation induction

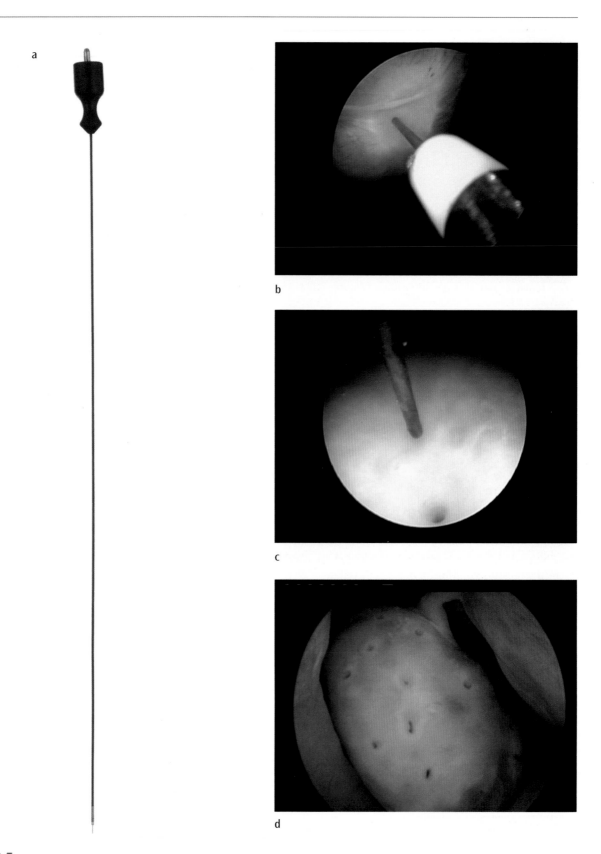

Figure 10.5
Drilling of the ovarian capsule using a 5 Fr bipolar needle (Karl Storz, Tüttlingen, Germany). (a) A 5 Fr bipolar needle. (b and c) The needle is placed perpendicular to the ovarian surface. (d) At the end of the procedure, approximately 10–15 small holes are made on the ovarian surface.

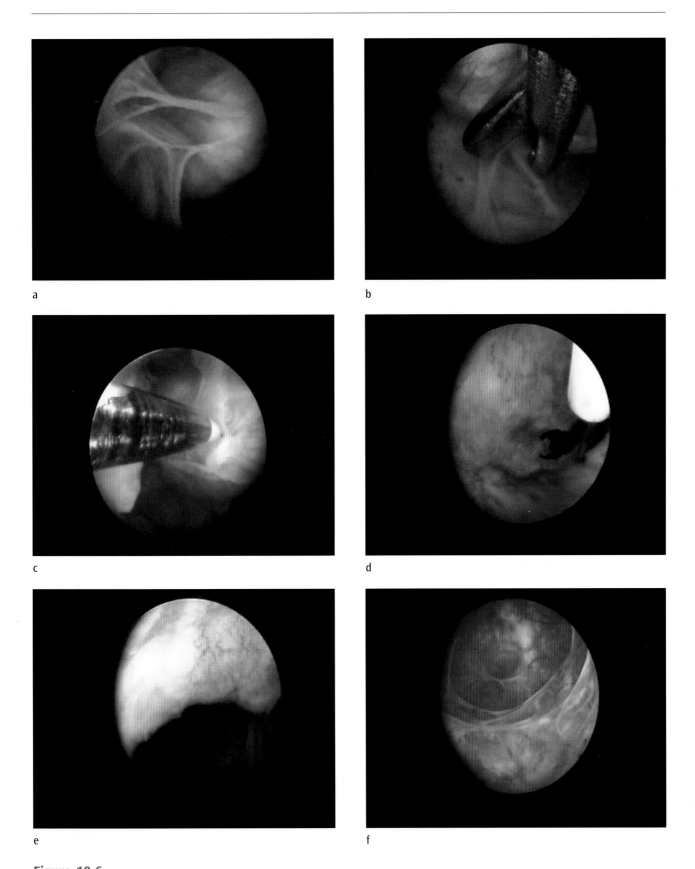

a

b

c

d

e

f

Figure 10.6
Adhesiolysis and opening of the hydrosalpinx using scissors and the bipolar coagulation and cutting needle. (a) The hydrosalpinx with adhesions. (b) Adhesiolysis using microscissors. (c and d) Opening the hydrosalpinx using the bipolar needle. (e and f) Introduction of a 2.9 mm endoscope with visualization of complete obstructed tubal lumen.

Table 10.1 Advantages and disadvantages of the vaginal approach in operative procedures

Advantages
- Direct access to Fallopian tubes, ovaries, fossa ovarica and posterior leaf of the broad ligament not requiring extra manipulation
- Watery distention medium keeps organs afloat and intestines at a distance
- Accurate identification of small superficial lesions
- Low morbidity

Disadvantages
- No panoramic view
- Limited to minor procedures
- Uncontrolled bleeding will blur the vision
- Contraindicated in acute situations (e.g. bleeding or infection)
- Still time consuming
- Training is mandatory

can be easier to perform, with reduced risks of ovarian hyperstimulation.

Easy performance and very low morbidity makes this procedure preferable over a long-lasting and sometimes difficult ovulation induction with a low-dose step-up protocol with gonadotropins and is certainly recommended before referral of patients to an in vitro fertilization (IVF) program.

Tubal reconstructive surgery

Using small scissors and the bipolar coagulation and cutting needle, adhesiolysis of tubo-ovarian adhesions can be performed. The use of pre-warmed Ringer's lactate as a distention medium provides a remarkable delineation between the different organs and the adhesions and offers the possibility for an accurate adhesiolysis and dissection. Also, in presence of hydrosalpinges, adhesiolysis allows the anatomical restoration of the tubo-ovarian relation. The site of invagination can be easily identified and the hydrosalpinx can be opened by performing an incision, as performed at previous microsurgical interventions (Figure 10.6). After opening the hydrosalpinx, the intratubal mucosal folds can be inspected through a salpingoscopy and the damage evaluated using the previously described classification system.[16–18] This way, patients can accurately and without delay be referred for microsurgical salpingostomy or IVF treatment. A technical advantage of transvaginal over transabdominal salpingoscopy is that the normal position of the ampullary segment lies in the axis of the scope. Consequently, salpingoscopy can be performed

without supplementary manipulation. The same 2.9 mm endoscope is used and distention of the ampullary segment is obtained through the continuous drip of Ringer's lactate.

Conclusion

Our experience shows the feasibility of using transvaginal access for the performance of well-defined limited operative procedures. In the absence of a panoramic view, major surgery is excluded, as is surgery in ever-acute situations such as intraperitoneal bleeding or infection. The direct access to the Fallopian tubes, ovaries, fossa ovarica, and posterior leaf of the broad ligament makes the technique very suitable for the treatment of superficial endometriosis and for drilling of the ovarian surface. The use of a watery distention medium keeps organs afloat and allows an accurate identification of small superficial lesions and a good delineation of the different structures. Because of the distention and the floating of the organs, the intestines are kept at a distance.

The low morbidity of the transvaginal procedure, in contrast with the pain experienced after SL due to irritation caused by the CO_2 pneumoperitoneum, has meant that procedures can be performed in a day hospital, with patients returning home the same day and getting back to work after 1 or 2 days.

Although organs are easy accessible, accurate identification and recognition of the anatomical situation is necessary to avoid unnecessary major complications.[19] Therefore, operative procedures should be reserved for those surgeons with enough experience gained with the diagnostic transvaginal laparoscopic procedures.

Our preliminary experience is promising, but has to be confirmed by larger series. The development of improved and adapted instrumentation will make surgical handling more accurate and less time consuming.

References

1. Gordts S, Campo R, Rombauts L, Brosens I. Transvaginal hydrolaparoscopy as an outpatient procedure for infertility investigation. Hum Reprod 1998; 13: 99–103.
2. Campo R, Gordts S, Rombauts L, Brosens I. Diagnostic accuracy of transvaginal hydrolaparoscopy in infertility. Fertil Steril 1999; 71: 1157–60.
3. Gordts S, Brosens I, Gordts S, Puttemans P, Campo R. Progress in transvaginal hydrolaparoscopy. Obstet Gynecol Clin North Am 2004; 31: 631–9, x.
4. Sampson JA. Peritoneal endometriosis due to the menstrual dissemination of endometrial tissues into the peritoneal cavity. Am J Obstet Gynecol 1927; 14: 442–69..
5. Hughesdon PE. The structure of endometrial cysts of the ovary. J Obstet Gynaecol Br Emp 1957; 64: 481–7.

6. Brosens IA, Puttemans PJ, Deprest J. The endoscopic localization of endometrial implants in the ovarian chocolate cyst. Fertil Steril 1994; 61: 1034–8.

7. Gordts S, Campo R, Brosens I. Experience with transvaginal hydrolaparoscopy for reconstructive tubo-ovarian surgery. Reprod Biomed Online 2002; 4 (Suppl 3): 72–5.

8. Gordts S, Boeckx W, Brosens I. Microsurgery of endometriosis in infertile patients. Fertil Steril 1984; 42: 520–5.

9. Brosens IA, Van Ballaer P, Puttemans P, Deprest J. Reconstruction of the ovary containing large endometriomas by an extraovarian endosurgical technique. Fertil Steril 1996; 66: 517–21.

10. Molinas CR, Tjwa M, Vanacker B et al. Role of CO_2 pneumoperitoneum-induced acidosis in CO_2 pneumoperitoneum-enhanced adhesion formation in mice. Fertil Steril 2004; 81: 708–11.

11. Elkelani OA, Molinas CR, Mynbaev O, Koninckx PR. Prevention of adhesions with crystalloids during laparoscopic surgery in mice. J Am Assoc Gynecol Laparosc 2002; 9: 447–52.

12. Elkelani OA, Binda MM, Molinas CR, Koninckx PR. Effect of adding more than 3% oxygen to carbon dioxide pneumoperitoneum on adhesion formation in a laparoscopic mouse model. Fertil Steril 2004; 82: 1616–22.

13. Casa A, Sesti F, Marziali M, Gulemi L, Piccione E. Transvaginal hydrolaparoscopic ovarian drilling using bipolar electrosurgery to treat anovulatory women with polycystic ovary syndrome. J Am Assoc Gynecol Laparosc 2003; 10: 219–22.

14. Fernandez H, Watrelot A, Alby JD et al. Fertility after ovarian drilling by transvaginal fertiloscopy for treatment of polycystic ovary syndrome. J Am Assoc Gynecol Laparosc 2004; 11: 374–8.

15. Heylen SM, Puttemans PJ, Brosens IA. Polycystic ovarian disease treated by laparoscopic argon laser capsule drilling: comparison of vaporization versus perforation technique. Hum Reprod 1994; 9: 1038–42.

16. De Bruyne F, Hucke J, Willers R. The prognostic value of salpingoscopy. Hum Reprod 1997; 12: 266–71.

17. Puttemans P, Brosens I, Delattin P, Vasquez G, Boeckx W. Salpingoscopy versus hysterosalpingography in hydrosalpinges. Hum Reprod 1987; 2: 535–40.

18. Gordts S, Campo R, Rombauts L, Brosens I. Transvaginal salpingoscopy: an office procedure for infertility investigation. Fertil Steril 1998; 70: 523–6.

19. Fernandez H. [Two complications of ovarian drilling by fertiloscopy; Gynecol Obstet Fertil 2003; 31: 844–6]. Gynecol Obstet Fertil 2004; 32: 265–6 [in French].

11

Cost-effectiveness of office transvaginal laparoscopy

Carolien AM Koks, Olga EAA van Tetering, Ben-Willem Mol, and Maarten AHM Wiegerinck

Introduction

In the assessment of a diagnostic procedure, not only clinical arguments such as diagnostic accuracy or patient safety but also economic aspects are of importance. There are several types of economic analysis available for the evaluation of health care technology.[1] In cost-effectiveness analysis, costs are related to the effect of a particular treatment. In fertility care, an acceptable measure for effectiveness is pregnancy or ongoing pregnancy. More recently, a shift has been made in which the effectiveness is expressed in terms of live birth rate.

Alternatives for cost-effectiveness analysis are cost-utility analysis or cost-benefit analysis. In cost-utility analysis, the outcome of medical interventions is expressed in utilities, e.g. life years that are adjusted for the quality of life of these years. Since in fertility care the outcome of interest is the birth of a healthy baby, cost-utility analysis is not a necessary or even appropriate technique. In cost-benefit analysis, not only the costs but also the potential benefits of interventions are expressed in financial terms. Since there is no uniform extrapolation of parents having a baby into financial terms, cost-benefit analysis is only rarely applied in fertility care. In this chapter, we will focus on cost-effectiveness rather than cost-benefit or cost-utility analysis.

How do we assess the cost-effectiveness of office transvaginal laparoscopy (TVL)? The effectiveness of a diagnostic procedure depends on the quality of diagnostic information obtained from this procedure and on the risk of procedure-related side effects or complications, the prevalence of a particular disease in the population in which the test is applied, and on the availability of an effective treatment in patients with the disease that the test under study is trying to detect.

If the side effects of a particular treatment are mild or if its costs are low, the consequences of a false-positive diagnosis, which would result in treatment of a person without the disease, are limited. If, however, a particular treatment generates severe side effects or if its costs are high, the consequences of a false-positive diagnosis are far more serious. Similarly, the consequences of a false-negative diagnosis are limited in case delay of the required treatment in a patient has a small impact on the outcome for the patient, whereas the consequences of a false-negative diagnosis are far more serious when delay of effective treatment affects the prognosis of the patient. Thus, the valuation of consequences of false-positive and false-negative test results has an impact on the value of a diagnostic test. Apart from the prevalence of disease and the performance of the test, the therapeutic context, i.e. benefits and harm of incorrect treatment and non-treatment, are of importance in the assessment of the value of the test. Furthermore, the costs and harm of the test itself affect the value of the test.

The fact that a diagnostic test can only become of value for the patient if it improves her health status, has consequences for test evaluation. Considering the therapeutic context, a diagnostic test reduces uncertainty on the disease status, thereby increasing the foundation for the decision to provide or withhold treatment. The aim of diagnostic testing is then to increase the probability of presence of disease in a subgroup of patients in such a way that the expected potential benefits of treatment outweigh the expected potential harm of treatment, or to decrease the probability of presence of disease in such a way that the expected potential benefit of non-treatment outweighs the expected potential harm of non-treatment.

Apart from its impact on therapeutic decisions, the information provided by diagnostic tests can also be of direct value for the patient. Patients may want to be informed about the cause of their disease or about their prognosis. For example, subfertile couples might be relieved once they know that the cause of their subfertility can be due to tubal damage. The assessment of this 'informative' value of a diagnostic test makes other demands on evaluation of diagnostic tests, which are beyond the scope of this chapter.[2]

Table 11.1 Quality of studies discussed in this chapter

Author	Year	Population	Number of patients	Selection bias	Verification bias	Blinding	Prospective	Consecutive patients	Unit of analysis
Shibahara[12]	2001	Women with primary or secondary subfertility, mean age 31.9 years (22–42 years), average subfertility period 3.6 years (1–10 years)	41	?	+	No	Yes	37	Tubes
Cicinelli[13]	2001	Subfertile women, mean age 29–30 years, average subfertility period 2.9–3.3 years	23	–	–	Yes	Yes	22	Patients
Fujiwara[16]	2003	Women with primary or secondary subfertility, mean age 31 years (23–42 years), average subfertility period 4.0 years (1.25–12.6 years)	36	+	+	No	No	36	Patients
Moore[7]	2001	Women with primary or secondary subfertility, failure to conceive 6 months after the HSG	10	+	+	No	No	10	Patients
Campo[17]	1999	Subfertile women with normal gynecologic examination	10	–	+	Yes	Yes	10	Tubes
Darai[18]	2000	Women with primary (n = 39) or secondary subfertility of more than 2 years, normal HSG, mean age 31 years (21–40 years)	60	+	+	Yes	Yes	54	Patients
Dechaud[19]	2001	Women with primary or secondary subfertility, normal HSG, mean age 33.5 years (26–40 years), mean duration of subfertility 36 months (24–180 months)	23	–	+	Yes	Yes	22	Patients
Nawroth[20]	2001	Women with primary (n = 31) or secondary subfertility >1 year, mean age 32 ± 4.3 years	43	–	+	No	Yes	40	Tubes
Casa[21]	2002	Women with unexplained primary subfertility >1 year, normal HSG, mean age 32.1 years (22–43 years)	60	–	+	Yes	Yes	54	Patients
Brosens[23]	2001	Multimember study, videotapes of women with minimal and mild endometriosis and unexplained subfertility	21	+	+	Yes	No	21	Patients

Table 11.2 Failure rate of transvaginal laparoscopy (TVL) in studies comparing TVL with hysterosalpingography (HSG)

Author	TVL	HSG
Shibahara[12]	3/41	1/41
Cicinelli[13]	1/23	0/23
Fujiwara[16]	0/36	0/36
Moore[7]	0/10	0/10
Campo[17]	0/10	0/10
Darai[18]	6/60	0/60
Dechaud[19]	1/23	0/23
Nawroth[20]	3/43	Not performed
Casa[21]	4/60	0/60
Brosens[23]	Not specified	Not specified
Total	18/306 = 5.9%	1/263 = 0.4%

In 1998, TVL was introduced as a new diagnostic outpatient procedure for exploration of the tubo-ovarian structures and tubal patency in infertile patients with no obvious pelvic pathology.[3] The procedure can be performed in an outpatient setting under local anesthesia. In addition, a diagnostic hysteroscopy can be performed with the same optic as the TVL. There is no need for an operating theater, general anesthesia, or a pneumoperitoneum, with its risk of drying and acidosis of the tissues, and the risk of severe injuries to the pelvic vessels is decreased.

Warmed saline is used as hydroflotation during TVL for inspection of the tubo-ovarian structures. With TVL, not only tubal patency but also periadnexal adhesions and endometriosis can be visualized. During the same procedure, a salpingoscopy can be performed.[4,5] The procedure can be followed on a video screen by the patient, and this allows it to be explained to her and her partner.

In cases of abnormal findings or incomplete evaluation by TVL, laparoscopy is indicated as a second step of evaluation.

In the years after its introduction, TVL was also introduced as an operative procedure for treatment of superficial endometriosis,[6–8] endometriotic cysts,[6] adhesions,[6–8] and for electrocoagulation of the ovaries in clomiphene citrate-resistant women.[6,9–11] Furthermore, a salpingostomy has been performed during TVL.[6]

Thusfar, the large majority of data on the accuracy and safety of this method come from the early adaptors of this technique. From their studies, it is concluded that this new diagnostic technique can be offered as an early investigation in the infertility work-up in an outpatient setting. However, the clinical value of TVL has not been evaluated in large cohort studies.

In this chapter, we will report on characteristics of TVL and of its competitors. We will discuss the clinical relevance and methodologic quality of each study (Table 11.1), and report on failure rate (Table 11.2), accuracy of diagnosing tubal occlusion (Table 11.3), adhesions (Table 11.4), and endometriosis (Table 11.5). We will focus successively on the capacity to predict pregnancy, on the side effects of the procedure, and on the costs.

Table 11.3 Diagnosis of unilateral and bilateral tubal occlusions

Author	TVL	HSG	Laparoscopy
Shibahara[12]	Not specified	Not specified	Not performed
Cicinelli[13]	6/22 unilateral occlusion 0/22 bilateral occlusion	7/22 unilateral occlusion 1/22 bilateral occlusion	Not performed
Fujiwara[16]	7/36	18/36 (10/36 unilateral, 6/36 bilateral, 2/36 stenosis)	Not performed
Moore[7]	1/10	1/10	Not performed
Campo[17]	Not specified	Not performed	Not specified
Darai[18]	13/54 tubal abnormalities	4/60 (tubal spasm)	14/54 tubal abnormalities
Dechaud[19]	0/22	0/23	0/23
Nawroth[20]	1/72 visible tubes	Not performed	1/80 tubes
Casa[21]	7/56	0/60	9/56
Brosens[23]	Not specified	Not performed	Not specified
Total	35/236 =14.8%	31/211 = 14.7%	24/173 = 13.9%

TVL, transvaginal laparoscopy; HSG, hysterosalpinography.

Table 11.4 Diagnosis of peritubal adhesions

Author	TVL	HSG	Laparoscopy
Shibahara[12]	22/68 tubes	0/68 tubes	Not performed
Cicinelli[13]	6/22 patients	6/22 patients	Not performed
Fujiwara[16]	23/36	6/36	Not performed
Moore[7]	2/10	0/10	Not performed
Campo[17]	12/19 tubes	Not performed	7/19 tubes
Darai[18]	10/54	0/54	15/54
Dechaud[19]	7/22 patients[a]	0/23	7/23 patients[b]
Nawroth[20]	1/40	Not performed	1/40
Casa[21]	11/56	0/60	15/56
Brosens[23]	12/21	Not performed	4/21
Total	106/348 (30%)	12/273 (4%)	49/213 (23%)

TVL, transvaginal laparoscopy; HSG, hysterosalpingography.
[a]3 patients also had endometriosis.
[b]6 patients also had endometriosis.

Table 11.5 Diagnosis of endometriosis

Author	TVL	HSG	Laparoscopy
Shibahara[12]	Not specified	Not specified	Not performed
Cicinelli[13]	2/22	0/22	Not performed
Fujiwara[16]	1/36	0/36	Not performed
Moore[7]	3/10	0/10	Not performed
Campo[17]	7/10	Not performed	7/10
Darai[18]	6/54	0/54	11/54
Dechaud[19]	5/22[a]	0/23	13/23[b]
Nawroth[20]	2/40	Not performed	10/40
Casa[21]	5/56	0/60 (56)	9/56
Brosens[23]	Not specified	Not performed	10/21
Total	31/250 (12.4%)	0/205 (0%)	60/204 (29.4%)

TVL, transvaginal laparoscopy; HSG, hysterosalpingography.
[a]3 patients also had adhesions.
[b]6 patients also had adhesions.

Diagnostic accuracy

Transvaginal endoscopy in comparison with other tubal tests

Studies comparing transvaginal laparoscopy with hysterosalpingography

In a retrospective study of Shibahara et al, the diagnostic findings at TVL were compared to findings at hysterosalpingography (HSG) in patients with and without past *Chlamydia trachomatis* infection.[12] The study population consisted of 41 patients with primary or secondary subfertility. The indication to perform a TVL were tubal obstruction and/or peritubal adhesions as suggested by the HSG, positive *C. trachomatis* antibody titer (CAT) testing, diagnosis of early-stage endometriosis, and unexplained subfertility. In three patients, access to the pouch of Douglas failed at TVL, whereas in one patient HSG could not be carried out. In 37 out of 41 patients, a comparison of HSG and TVL could be made. For the diagnosis of tubal patency, there was no significant difference in the discrepancy rates between HSG and TVL in women with and without past *C. trachomatis* infection. However, in 14 (58.3%) of 24 tubes from 14 patients with past *C. trachomatis* infection, peritubal adhesions were diagnosed by TVL and not by HSG.

In the group of women without the infection, only eight (18.2%) out of 44 tubes of 23 women showed peritubal adhesions at TVL. There was a significant difference in the discrepancy rates of the diagnosis of peritubal adhesions between HSG and TVL in the two groups ($p = 0.0007$).

Cicinelli et al performed a randomized controlled trial comparing HSG on the one hand and TVL with diagnostic hysteroscopy on the other hand in 23 subfertile women without obvious pelvic pathology.[13] The ages of the patients ranged between 25 and 34 years and all women had been unable to conceive for at least 1 year. All women had natural ovulatory cycles and normal findings for both transvaginal ultrasound examination and cervical bacterial cultures. The diagnostic agreement between these procedures with respect to tubal patency and uterine cavity abnormality was evaluated. The order of the two tests was determined randomly. In one patient there was no entrance to the peritoneal cavity. With respect to tubal patency, in 95% (21/22) of the cases findings at TVL were in accordance with HSG (15 patients with bilateral patency and six patients with a unilateral tubal obstruction). In one case TVL showed bilateral patency whereas HSG diagnosed an intramural obstruction of both Fallopian tubes. Endometriosis was detected in two cases during TVL.

The agreement between TVL and HSG in the diagnosis of intrauterine pathology was poor (43%). A normal uterine cavity was diagnosed in 10 cases and uterine malformation in three cases by both HSG and hysteroscopy. In nine cases where HSG showed a normal uterine cavity, hysteroscopy diagnosed endometrial polyps ($n = 6$) and endometritis ($n = 3$). However, the impact of these minor intrauterine abnormalities on subfertility was the subject of two earlier studies and both studies concluded that treatment of small polyps, <2 cm, did not increase pregnancy rates in in vitro fertilization (IVF) cycles.[14,15]

In a retrospective study of Fujiwara et al, TVL was performed in 36 women with suspected tubal subfertility and HSG findings or subfertility of unknown etiology.[16] Complete visualization of both adnexa was achieved in 67 of 72 adnexa (93.1%), whereas adhesions caused incomplete visualization in five other cases. Discrepancies between TVL and HSG for patency and peritubal adhesions were observed in 16.4% (11 of 67 tubes) and 25.4% of adnexa (17 of 67 adnexa), respectively. Findings not identified on HSG, such as fimbrial or tubal deformity, were present at TVL in 13% of adnexa. Endometriosis was observed during TVL in only one case.

In a retrospective study of Moore et al, 10 patients had an HSG (months) before TVL.[7] There was 100% concordance with respect to tubal pathology (nine patients with bilateral patent tubes and one patient with unilateral tubal occlusion) However at TVL, in five (56%) of the nine women with bilateral patent tubes, endometriosis (three women) or adhesions (two women) was diagnosed.

Transvaginal endoscopy compared with diagnostic laparoscopy

Diagnostic laparoscopy is still considered as the reference standard to investigate tuboperitoneal disease. The first studies on TVL were prospective comparisons to assess the feasibility and accuracy of TVL compared with diagnostic laparoscopy in subfertile women.[3,17] Different operators evaluated the findings of the two procedures. In order to evaluate the accuracy of TVL, findings in terms of tubal pathology, endometriosis, and adhesions were analyzed.

In their first study, Gordts et al performed a diagnostic laparoscopy with dye testing after TVL in 7 patients.[3] The results were comparable, but for filmy adhesions that were more often seen during TVL. In a later study by the same group, diagnostic laparoscopy with dye testing and TVL were performed by two independent investigators in 10 subfertile women without obvious pelvic pathology.[17] Ovarian adhesions were more frequently found during TVL (63%) than during diagnostic laparoscopy with dye testing (37%). This difference may be due to the fact that non-connecting adhesions are frequently seen during TVL. However, the clinical significance of these non-connecting adhesions is not known. There was complete agreement in the diagnosis of hydrosalpinges and endometriosis in both diagnostic procedures.

In a prospective comparative blinded study by Darai et al, TVL was performed in 60 patients immediately prior to a diagnostic laparoscopy with dye testing.[18] The inclusion criteria were subfertility of at least 2 years, normal ovulation, and normal gynecologic and ultrasonographic examination. All patients had an HSG performed before entering the study, and all HSGs were considered as normal except for four cases in which tubal spasms were suspected. Different operators who were not aware of the initial findings of TVL performed the standard laparoscopy. Failed entry occurred in 10% of patients. Overall, findings at TVL were closely related to the findings at diagnostic laparoscopy in 49 out of 54 cases (90.7%). In cases of complete evaluation at TVL, the sensitivity and specificity values were 92.3% and 100%, respectively.

Dechaud et al performed TVL immediately prior to standard laparoscopy in a prospective comparative study.[19] The laparoscopist was never aware of the findings at TVL. Both procedures were performed under general anesthesia. Twenty-three subfertile patients with at least 2 years of unexplained subfertility and normal findings at HSG were included in this study. In 41% of cases, the TVL revealed a normal pelvic examination confirmed by laparoscopy. Among the nine patients in whom TVL showed pathologic findings, there were no normal laparoscopies. Conversely, pathologic laparoscopies were found in four of the 14 normal TVLs. In all those four patients, endometriosis (three rAFS1 and one rAFS2 [revised American Fertility Society]) was diagnosed during diagnostic laparoscopy. Overall sensitivity was 70%, for a specificity of 100%.

Another prospective comparing study on TVL vs diagnostic laparoscopy was performed by Nawroth et al.[20] The study comprised 43 subfertile women with subfertility of more than 1 year, ovulatory cycles as well as inconspicuous gynecologic and sonographic examination. There was complete agreement between laparoscopy and TVL in the diagnosis of tubal occlusion and adhesions. For the diagnosis of endometriosis, the sensitivity was 100%, for a specificity of 20%.

Casa et al also performed a prospective blinded study to assess TVL in comparison with diagnostic laparoscopy.[21] Sixty patients with unexplained subfertility of at least 1 year and normal findings on gynecologic examination, normal ultrasound examination, and normal HSG were included. All procedures were performed under general anesthesia. Seven of the nine (77.8%) tubal abnormalities and five of nine cases of endometriosis (55.5%) were correctly diagnosed by TVL. In the cases of missed diagnosis (two tubal abnormalities, four endometriosis), severe pelvic adhesions prevented complete evaluation. There were no false-positive results by TVL. If false-negative findings are calculated only in cases of complete evaluation by TVL, both sensitivity and specificity values were 100%.

In a study of Gordts et al, 29 of 149 (19%) patients underwent an operative laparoscopy based on the findings of TVL. The diagnosis of endometriosis and tubo-ovarian adhesions was confirmed at the laparoscopy. However, more adhesions were diagnosed at TVL.[22]

In a retrospective multicenter (five centers) trial, the same investigators viewed videotapes of standard laparoscopy and TVL by independent observers in random order.[23] Forty-three subfertile patients with negative findings on gynecologic investigation and vaginal sonography who were scheduled for diagnostic laparoscopy as part of their fertility investigation were enrolled in this study. The videotapes of transvaginal hydrolaparoscopy and standard laparoscopy were considered conclusive if all surfaces of both ovaries were visualized. Four videotapes of standard laparoscopy and nine tapes of transvaginal hydrolaparoscopy were considered inconclusive. Minimal and mild endometriosis and unexplained infertility were diagnosed at standard laparoscopy in 10 and 11 patients, respectively. These patients were included in the study. In patients with minimal and mild endometriosis or unexplained subfertility, TVL showed adhesions more often than laparoscopy (12/21 vs 4/21).

We are not aware of studies in the literature comparing microlaparoscopy and TVL for exploration of the tubo-ovarian structures

Other tests

Accuracy of hysterosalpingography

The accuracy of HSG in the diagnoses of tubal occlusion and peritubal adhesions using laparoscopy with chromo-pertubation as the reference standard has been assessed in a meta-analysis.[24]

This meta-analysis incorporated 20 studies comparing HSG and laparoscopy. For tubal occlusion, the reported sensitivity and specificity differed between studies. In a subset of three studies that evaluated HSG and laparoscopy independently, a point-estimate of 65% for sensitivity (95% CI 50–78%) and 83% for specificity (95% CI 77–88%) was calculated. For peritubal adhesions, a summary ROC (receiver operating characteristic) curve could be estimated that indicated a poor diagnostic performance of HSG in the diagnosis of tubal adhesions. The authors concluded that the performance of HSG in the diagnosis of tubal occlusion is sufficient for its use as a triage before laparoscopy and, that after a normal HSG, laparoscopy can be withheld for a considerable time. HSG was not reliable for the evaluation of peritubal adhesions.

Accuracy of *Chlamydia* antibody titer screening

The discriminative capacity of *C. trachomatis* antibody in the diagnosis of any tubal pathology was analyzed in another meta-analysis.[25] This meta-analysis incorporated 23 studies comparing CAT and laparoscopy for tubal pathology. The diagnostic performance of CAT depended on the type of assay that was used. Summary ROC curves of studies using enzyme-linked immunosorbent assay (ELISA) or (micro)-immunofluorescence (MIF/IF) revealed a better discrimination than the summary ROC curve of immunoperoxidase assay (IPA). The summary ROC curves for ELISA and MIF revealed a discriminative capacity that was comparable to that of HSG. The performance of CAT by means of ELISA, MIF, or IF in the diagnosis of any tubal pathology is therefore sufficient to consider its use as a triage before further testing for tubal disease.

In view of the data presented in this section, we feel that at present it is not conclusive how the accuracy of TVL compares with its main competitors, i.e. HSG, CAT, or laparoscopy. The failure rate of TVL in these comparative studies was 5.9%, which was clearly higher than the 0.4% that was calculated for HSG. However, in later larger studies in which the investigators were more experienced in performing TVL, the failure rate tends to be less (3.5%).[26] The studies in which TVL was compared with HSG or laparoscopy in identical patients had too little power to draw definite conclusions. However, the number of patients in whom tubal occlusion was diagnosed was virtually similar for the three groups, with 14.8%, 14.7%, and 13.9% for TVL, HSG, and laparoscopy, respectively (see Table 11.3).

Endometriosis was not diagnosed at HSG, but was identified in 12% of the TVL procedures and 29% of the laparoscopy procedures. It remains controversial as to whether this minimal and mild endometriosis (rAFS I and II) has an influence on infertility and whether or not operative therapy would improve the fertility. The study of Marcoux et al showed that electrocoagulation of minimal and mild endometriosis could improve fecundity, but in a small study of Parazinni there was not a significant difference in fecundity after resection or ablation of visible endometriosis in women with minimal and mild endometriosis, leaving this subject controversial.[27,28]

Peritubal adhesions were detected in 4% of the HSGs, 22% of the diagnostic laparoscopies, and even in 30% of the TVLs. However, it is unknown whether these adhesions have negative consequences for fertility prospects, or whether treatment of these adhesions is useful. The study of Collins et al indicated that the impact of peritubal adhesions was very limited.[29]

Prognostic capacity

Prognostic capacity of transvaginal laparoscopy

In a small retrospective study of Fujiwara et al that we discussed earlier in this chapter, the prognostic capacity for the occurrence of treatment-independent pregnancy of TVL was evaluated.[16] On the basis of findings of TVL and HSG, expectant management, artificial insemination, and assisted reproductive technology (ART) were indicated in eight (22.2%), 15 (41.7%), and 13 (36.1%) of the 36 patients, respectively. High pregnancy rates were observed after TVL, especially in the expectant management group (seven of eight women, 87.5%). The mean duration of unprotected intercourse of these women was 47.6 months, and mean period after TVL until pregnancy was only 6.0 months (3–12 months). Three of these patients had bilateral tubal patency on TVL, whereas HSG suggested the presence of fimbrial adhesions and tubal stenosis. Seven of the 15 (46.7%) women who were treated with artificial insemination became pregnant. In five of these seven patients, discrepancies in findings with HSG were observed. In three of the five patients, HSG and TVL both revealed unilateral obstruction, but TVL also confirmed normal morphology and patency of the contralateral side. In the other two patients, TVL diagnosed normal findings, whereas HSG suggested the presence of peritubal adhesions and tubal obstruction. Four of the seven pregnancies occurred after the first artificial insemination procedure. In three of these patients who became pregnant, discrepancies between HSG and TVL were observed, with normal findings on HSG in two of the three women, whereas TVL revealed the presence of severe fimbrial adhesions. In the

third patient, TVL revealed marked deformity of the tubal fimbria, which appeared normal on HSG. In this study, TVL seemed to be a useful and feasible procedure in selecting a further treatment strategy.

Prognostic capacity of hysterosalpingography and laparoscopy

The prognostic significance of HSG for fertility outcome has been evaluated in several cohort studies.[30,31]

In a cohort study from Amsterdam, consecutive patients undergoing HSG for subfertility between May 1985 and November 1987 were included in a retrospective study. Follow-up ended when pregnancy or tubal surgery occurred, or at the day of last contact. Kaplan–Meier curves for the occurrence of spontaneous intrauterine pregnancy (IUP) were constructed for a normal HSG, an HSG with a one-sided abnormality, and an HSG with a two-sided abnormality. Fecundity rate ratios (FRR) were calculated to express the association between HSG findings and the occurrence of spontaneous IUP. Of the 359 patients analyzed, 231 (64%) showed no tubal pathology on HSG, 67 (19%) had one-sided tubal pathology, and 61 (17%) had two-sided tubal pathology. The adjusted FRRs were 0.81 (95% CI 0.47–1.4) for one-sided pathology and 0.30 (95% CI 0.13–0.71) for two-sided pathology. Correction for informative censoring and sensitivity analysis did not alter these results. One-sided tubal pathology detected on HSG limits the fertility prospects only slightly, whereas two-sided tubal pathology detected on HSG reduces fertility prospects considerably.

In a prospective cohort study in 11 clinics participating in the Canadian Infertility Treatment Evaluation Study (CITES), consecutive couples who registered for the evaluation of subfertility and who underwent HSG and laparoscopy were included. Unilateral and bilateral tubal occlusion at HSG and laparoscopy were related to treatment-independent pregnancy. Cox regression was used to calculate FRRs for the occurrence of ongoing pregnancy. Of the 794 patients that were included, 114 (14%) showed one-sided tubal occlusion and 194 (24%) showed two-sided tubal occlusion on HSG. At laparoscopy, 94 (12%) showed one-sided tubal occlusion and 96 (12%) showed two-sided tubal occlusion. Occlusion detected on HSG and laparoscopy showed a moderate agreement beyond chance (weighted kappa-value = 0.42). Multivariate analysis showed FRRs of 0.80 and 0.49 for one-sided and two-sided tubal occlusion, respectively. For laparoscopy, these FRRs were 0.51 and 0.15, respectively. After a normal HSG or an HSG with one-sided tubal occlusion, laparoscopy showed two-sided occlusion in 5% of the patients, and fertility prospects in these patients were virtually zero. If two-sided tubal occlusion was detected on HSG but not during laparoscopy, fertility prospects were slightly impaired. Fertility prospects after a two-sided occluded HSG were strongly impaired in case laparoscopy showed one-sided and two-sided occlusion, with FRRs of 0.38 and 0.19, respectively.

This study showed that, although laparoscopy performed better than HSG as a predictor of future fertility, it should not be considered as the perfect test in the diagnosis of tubal pathology. For clinical practice, laparoscopy can be delayed after normal HSG for at least 10 months, since the probability that laparoscopy will show tubal occlusion after a normal HSG was very low.

The transvaginal laparoscopy procedure at our department

Since 1999, the TVL procedure has been performed in our clinic by three gynecologists with a special interest in reproductive medicine or by registrars under the supervision of one of these gynecologists. Apart from the first seven procedures, all procedures were performed at the outpatient clinic under local anesthesia. During the first year, some of the women undergoing a TVL had already had an HSG, and the TVL procedure was proposed instead of a diagnostic laparoscopy. Later, TVL was used as a first-line tubal investigation, replacing HSG.

All patients undergoing a TVL at the outpatient clinic are given oral and written information about the procedure. The procedure is scheduled in the proliferative phase of the menstrual cycle. Patients are premedicated with two tablets of bisacodyl, a mild rectal laxative, and Naprosyn (naproxen). Immediately before the procedure, an injection of 0.5 mg atropine is given intramuscularly. One year ago we decided only to give the mild rectal laxative, since we think that a full rectum gives a greater chance of causing a bowel injury instead of the small intestines. We also abandoned the atropine injection and have not had vasovagal events. A prophylactic dose of 1000 mg azithromycin is given when there is a positive CAT or when serious tubal pathology is diagnosed during the procedure.

The procedure is performed with the patient in the dorsal gynecologic position. After insertion of a Trelat speculum, the vagina is disinfected with aqueous chlorhexidine solution. The central part of the posterior cervix is infiltrated with 1–2 ml of Ultracaine (articaine). A tenaculum is placed on the posterior cervix and a balloon catheter is put in the uterine cavity and the balloon inflated with 1–2 ml of air for the chromoperturbation. Local anesthesia with 2–3 ml of Ultracaine is performed in the vaginal vault, 1–2 cm below the cervix. A small incision is made at this place and a specially designed trocar system (Circon ACMI, Stamford, CA, USA) is introduced. The system consists of an adapted Verres needle 25 cm in length, a dilatating device, and a trocar 3.9 mm in outside diameter. All three parts fit together, but the Verres needle is 15 mm longer than the dilatating device. The Verres needle is inserted briskly to avoid tenting of the peritoneum. Progressively, the dilator and trocar are inserted transvaginally into the pouch of Douglas, after which the dilator and Verres needle are removed and replaced by a rigid 2.7 mm wide-angle optical system, which is placed in the 3.9 mm shaft system ensuring irrigation during the procedure. Continuous infusion with saline solution at 37°C is then started.

After infusion of saline and some orientation, the investigation starts at the posterior uterine wall. Then the scope is moved laterally to identify the tubo-ovarian structures. The ovarian surface is inspected, from the ligamentum ovarium propium going to the fossa ovarica and the dorsal part of the ovary. The fimbrial part of the Fallopian tubes are inspected as well as the tubo-ovarian contact. Then a dye test is performed to test the patency of the tube. The contralateral side is inspected in the same way. Throughout the whole procedure, irrigation with warm saline is continued, keeping the bowel and the tubo-ovarian structures afloat.

After the procedure, the fluid is removed from the abdomen through the trocar. The puncture site in the fornix posterior is not sutured unless there is active bleeding. At our department an additional hysteroscopy is only performed in case of suspected uterine anomaly or intrauterine pathology, or in case of tubal pathology. After the procedure, women are asked to rate the experienced pain on a visual analogue scale (VAS) from 0 (no pain) to 10 (unbearable pain). The acceptability of the procedure is also rated on the same VAS from 0 to 10.

Patients are informed that some vaginal leakage or bleeding can occur, and are advised not to use vaginal tampons. The patient leaves the outpatient clinic immediately after the procedure.

Results and prognostic capacity of our transvaginal laparoscopy procedures

In the period from 1999 until 2004 a total of 284 TVLs were performed. For the follow-up study, women were followed until pregnancy or for at most 12 months. We registered the start of treatment, intrauterine insemination (IUI), or IVF and occurrence of pregnancy (ongoing, ectopic pregnancy, and miscarriage) with or without treatment. Findings at TVL were related to time to ongoing pregnancy using Cox proportional hazards analysis. For the purpose of the analysis, spontaneous pregnancies and pregnancies after IUI were considered as successes, whereas pregnancies after IVF were considered to be failures.

Of these 284 women, 236 women had a follow-up period of 12 months. In 226/236 (95.7%) of the patients, access to the pouch of Douglas was achieved and adnexa could be visualized. Among the failures, there were two cases of rectal perforation: one perforation occurred in a woman with a mobile but retroverted uterus; the other rectal perforation occurred in a patient with a distended rectum. Both women were treated expectantly and received antibiotics for 7 days. In 147 (65%) of these 226 women, normal tubo-ovarian structures with patent tubes were visualized. In 35 women (16%), one of the tubes showed patency, the other obstructed or not visualized. Adhesions and endometriosis were diagnosed in 34 (15%), whereas serious tubal pathology was observed in 10 (4%) of the 226 women. There were six (2.1%) complications. Apart from the two patients with rectal perforation mentioned above, three bleedings at the puncture site, of which two stopped after local pressure, and one needed to be stitched, occurred. One of the patients was readmitted because of pain and a suspected pelvic infection. She received antibiotics and recovery was uneventful. VAS scores were 4.4 for pain and 1.8 for acceptability.

In women with two patent tubes without other pelvic pathology, the 12 months cumulative pregnancy rate was 54%. The presence of endometriosis and/or adhesions, as well as the presence of one patent tube had no impact on the fertility prospects (RR [relative risk] = 1.3 and 0.95, respectively). In case of serious tubal pathology, none of the patients conceived without treatment.

Decision analysis

The cost-effectiveness of strategies that can be used to detect tubal pathology in subfertile couples with respect to live birth rates, number of cycles of in vitro fertilization–embryo transfer (IVF-ET), and total costs has been assessed previously.[32] In this analysis, baseline characteristics of >2000 subfertile couples collected in the CITES were used. Expectant management, i.e. no diagnosis or treatment, was considered to be the reference strategy. In strategy 2 and 3, IVF-ET was either offered immediately or after 2.5 years. In strategy 4, the decision to offer or delay treatment was based on the spontaneous conception chances of the couple, based on female age, duration of subfertility, previous pregnancies, and regularity of the menstrual cycle. Moreover, nine strategies were evaluated incorporating combinations of CAT, cancer antigen 125 (CA-125) measurement, HSG, and laparoscopy. For each strategy, we calculated expected live birth rates, expected number of IVF-ET cycles, and expected total costs.

Expected spontaneous live birth rates were obtained from CITES. Expected IVF-ET success rates were obtained from a cohort study in the UK.

Without treatment, the 3-year expected cumulative live birth rate was 13%, whereas it varied between 34% and 49% for other strategies. Costs of these strategies varied between US$19 800 and US$27 500 per couple. The strategy in which the decision to perform laparoscopy either immediately or after 1 year, depending on the result of CAT, was the most cost-effective strategy, whereas the strategy in which this decision was based on the result of HSG was almost as cost-effective. Sensitivity analysis showed that the strategy starting with CAT was the most cost-effective in couples in which 3-year conception chances were >14%, whereas the strategy starting with HSG was the most cost-effective in couples with worse fertility prospects. Use of serum CA-125 measurement was only cost-effective in the case where fertility prospects were very poor.

The diagnostic work-up to detect tubal pathology in subfertile couples should start with CAT in couples with relatively good fertility prospects, whereas couples with relatively poor fertility prospects benefit from a strategy starting with immediate HSG.

Costs of transvaginal laparoscopy

In that analysis,[32] the costs of HSG and laparoscopy were US$100 and US$800, respectively. Table 11.6 shows the resources that are needed for HSG, laparoscopy, and TVL. As can be seen from the table, the amount of manpower needed for laparoscopy is more than for HSG and TVL, which both require approximately equal human resources. The main difference in costs between TVL and HSG will be due to differences in equipment. In the absence of formal cost studies on TVL, we estimate the costs of TVL to be between US$200 and US$300.

Conclusions

From the data presented in this chapter, we feel there is insufficient evidence to draw firm and crisp conclusions about the cost-effectiveness of TVL. In view of its lower costs, less risk on serious complications, and in view of the fact that TVL can be performed in an outpatient setting, TVL is potentially more attractive than laparoscopy. By performing TVLs, several investigators concluded that laparoscopies were avoided in 72%,[22] or could be avoided in 45%,[18] 41%,[19] and 46.2%,[5] of patients because of normal findings at TVL, which is an alternative option to laparoscopy in 41–72% of subfertile women undergoing

Table 11.6 Comparison of manpower and equipment for TVL, laparoscopy, and HSG

	TVL	Laparoscopy	HSG
Manpower			
Nurse day care unit	No	Yes	No
Transport to and from theater	No	Yes	No
Anesthesiologist	0	1	0
Assistant anesthesiologist	0	1	0
Theater nurse (2)	0	2	0
Nurse recovery unit	No	Yes	No
Assistant OPD	1	0	0
Gynecologist	1	1	1
Radiologist	0	0	1
Assistant radiologist	0	0	1
Procedure time	20 minutes	30 minutes	20 minutes
Duration stay in hospital	30 minutes	>6 hours	45 minutes
Hospital bed	No	Yes	No
Equipment			
Sterile covers	Yes	Yes	No
Speculum, tenaculum	Yes	Yes	Yes
Intrauterine balloon/catheter	Yes	Yes	Yes
Camera–light–monitor unit	Yes	Yes	No
Radiology unit	No	No	Yes

TVL, transvaginal laparoscopy; HSG, hysterosalpingography; OPD, outpatient department.

tubal investigation. However, more data from large multicenter clinical studies are needed before a clear preference for one of the diagnostic strategies discussed above can be expressed.

References

1. Gold MR, Siegel JE, Russel LB, Weinstein MB. Cost-Effectiveness in Health and Medicine. New York: Oxford University Press, 1996.
2. Asch DA, Patton JP, Hershey JC. Knowing for the sake of knowing: the value of prognostic information. Med Decis Making 1990; 10: 47–57.
3. Gordts S, Campo R, Rombauts L et al. Transvaginal hydrolaparoscopy as an outpatient procedure for infertility investigation. Hum Reprod 1998; 13: 99–103.
4. Gordts S, Campo R, Rombauts L et al. Transvaginal salpingoscopy: an office procedure for infertility investigation. Fertil Steril 1998; 70: 523–6.
5. Watrelot A, Dreyfus JM, Andine JP. Evaluation of the performance of fertiloscopy in 160 consecutive infertile patients with no obvious pathology. Hum Reprod 1999; 14: 707–11.
6. Gordts S, Campo R, Brosens I. Experience with transvaginal hydrolaparoscopy for reconstructive tubo-ovarian surgery. Reprod Biomed Online 2001; 4(3): 72–5.
7. Moore LM, Cohen BS. Diagnostic and operative transvaginal hydrolaparoscopy for infertility and pelvic pain. J Am Assoc Gynecol Laparosc 2001; 8(3): 393–7.
8. Moore LM, Cohen M, Liu GY. Experience with 109 cases of transvaginal laparoscopy. J Am Assoc Gynecol Laparosc 2003; 10(2): 282–5.
9. Fernandez H, Alby JD, Gervaise A et al. Operative transvaginal hydrolaparoscopy for treatment of polycystic ovary syndrome: a new minimally invasive surgery. Fertil Steril 2001; 75(3): 607–11.
10. Casa A, Sesti F, Marziali M et al. Transvaginal hydrolaparoscopic ovarian drilling using bipolar electrosurgery to treat anovulatory women with polycystic ovary syndrome. Am Assoc Gynecol Laparosc 2003; 10(2): 219–22.
11. Fernandez H, Watrelot A, Alby JD et al. Fertility after ovarian drilling by transvaginal fertiloscopy for treatment of polycystic ovary syndrome. J Am Assoc Gynecol Laparosc 2004; 11(3): 374–8.
12. Shibahara H, Fujiwara H, Hirano Y et al. Usefulness of transvaginal hydrolaparoscopy in investigating infertile women with *Chlamydia trachomatis* infection. Hum Reprod 2001; 16: 1690–3.
13. Cicinelli E, Matteo M, Causio F et al. Tolerability of the mini-pan-endoscopic approach (transvaginal hydrolaparoscopy and minihysteroscopy) versus hysterosalpingography in an outpatient infertility investigation. Fertil Steril 2001; 76(5): 1048–51.
14. Mastrominas M, Pistofidis GA, Dimitropoulus K. Fertility outcome after outpatient hysteroscopic removal of endometrial polyps and submucous fibroids. J Am Assoc Gynecol Laparosc 1996; 3(4 Suppl): S29.
15. Lass A, Williams G, Abusheika N et al. The effect of endometrial polyps on outcomes of in vitro fertilization (IVF) cycles. J Assist Reprod Genet 1999; 16(8): 410–15.
16. Fujiwara H, Shibahara H, Hirano Y et al. Usefulness and prognostic value of transvaginal hydrolaparoscopy in infertile women. Fertil Steril 2003; 79(1): 186–9.
17. Campo R, Gordts S, Rombauts L et al. Diagnostic accuracy of transvaginal hydrolaparoscopy in infertility. Fertil Steril 1999; 71: 1157–60.
18. Darai E, Dessolle L, Lecuru F et al. Transvaginal hydrolaparoscopy compared with laparoscopy for the evaluation of infertile women: a prospective comparative blind study. Hum Reprod 2000; 15: 2379–82.
19. Dechaud H, Ahmed SA, Aligier N et al. Does transvaginal hydrolaparoscopy render standard diagnostic laparoscopy obsolete for unexplained infertility investigation? Eur J Obstet Gynecol 2001; 94: 97–102.
20. Nawroth F, Foth D, Schmidt T et al. Results of a prospective comparative study of transvaginal hydrolaparoscopy and chromolaparoscopy in the diagnostics of infertility. Gynecol Obstet Invest 2001; 52: 184–8.
21. Casa A, Francesco S, Marziali M et al. Transvaginal hydrolaparoscopy vs. conventional laparoscopy for evaluating unexplained primary infertility in women. J Reprod Med 2002; 47(8): 617–20.
22. Gordts S, Campo R, Brosens I. Office transvaginal hydrolaparoscopy for early diagnosis of pelvic endometriosis and adhesions. J Am Assoc Gynecol Laparosc 2000; 7(1): 45–9.
23. Brosens I, Gordts S, Campo R. Transvaginal hydrolaparoscopy but not standard laparoscopy reveals subtle endometriotic adhesions of the ovary. Fertil Steril 2001; 75(5): 1009–12.
24. Swart P, Mol BWJ, Van der Veen F et al. The accuracy of hysterosalpingography in the diagnosis of tubal pathology, a meta-analysis. Fertil Steril 1995; 64: 486–91.
25. Mol BWJ, Dijkman AB, Wertheim P et al. The accuracy of chlamydia antibodies in the diagnosis of tubal pathology; a meta-analysis. Fertil Steril 1997; 67: 1031–7.

26. Gordts S, Brosens I, Gordts S et al. Progress in transvaginal hydrolaparoscopy. Obstet Gynecol Clin N Am 2004; 31: 631–9.

27. Marcoux S, Maheux R, Berube S. Laparoscopic surgery in infertile women with minimal or mild endometriosis. Canadian Collaborative Group on Endometriosis. N Engl J Med 1997; 337(4): 217–22.

28. Parazzini F. Ablation of lesions or no treatment in minimal-mild endometriosis in infertile women: a randomized trial. Gruppo Italiano per Lo Studio dell'Endometriosi. Hum Reprod 1999; 14(5): 1332–4.

29. Collins JA, Burrows EA, Willan AR. The prognosis for live birth among untreated infertile couples. Fertil Steril 1995; 64: 22–8.

30. Mol BWJ, Swart P, Bossuyt PMM et al. Is hysterosalpingography an important tool in predicting fertility outcome? Fertil Steril 1997; 67: 663–9.

31. Mol BWJ, Collins JA, Burrows EA et al. Comparison of hysterosalpingography and laparoscopy in predicting fertility outcome. Hum Reprod 1999; 14: 1737–42.

32. Mol BWJ, Collins JA, Van der Veen F et al. Cost-effectiveness analysis of hysterosalpingography, laparoscopy, and Chlamydia antibody testing in subfertile couples. Fertil Steril 2001; 75: 571–80.

Index